AF203056

## About the Author

**Peter Y. Chen**, PhD, was awarded a doctoral degree in 1991 from the University of South Florida with a major in industrial and organizational psychology. He is a professor of psychology at Auburn University, a fellow of the Society for Industrial and Organizational Psychology, past editor of the *Journal of Occupational Health Psychology*, and past president of the Society for Occupational Health Psychology. He has published more than 100 articles and two books, and his work has been cited over 10,000 times. One of his articles was deemed one of the eight most influential papers in the *Journal of Organizational Behavior*. In addition, he was ranked 29th among the most-cited authors between 2000 and 2004, in 30 management journals. The overarching aim of his research is to understand the process of change at the individual, organizational, community, and industry levels, and to develop ways to facilitate changes, with the goal of building a healthy workplace and society.

## Advances in Psychotherapy – Evidence-Based Practice

### Series Editor

**Danny Wedding**, PhD, MPH, Professor Emeritus, University of Missouri–Saint Louis, MO

### Associate Editors

**Jonathan S. Comer**, PhD, Professor of Psychology and Psychiatry, Director of Mental Health Interventions and Technology (MINT) Program, Center for Children and Families, Florida International University, Miami, FL

**J. Kim Penberthy**, PhD, ABPP, Professor of Psychiatry & Neurobehavioral Sciences, University of Virginia, Charlottesville, VA

**Kenneth E. Freedland**, PhD, Professor of Psychiatry and Psychology, Washington University School of Medicine, St. Louis, MO

**Linda C. Sobell**, PhD, ABPP, Professor, Center for Psychological Studies, Nova Southeastern University, Ft. Lauderdale, FL

The basic objective of this series is to provide therapists with practical, evidence-based treatment guidance for the most common disorders seen in clinical practice – and to do so in a reader-friendly manner. Each book in the series is both a compact "how-to" reference on a particular disorder for use by professional clinicians in their daily work and an ideal educational resource for students as well as for practice-oriented continuing education.

The most important feature of the books is that they are practical and easy to use: All are structured similarly and all provide a compact and easy-to-follow guide to all aspects that are relevant in real-life practice. Tables, boxed clinical "pearls," marginal notes, and summary boxes assist orientation, while checklists provide tools for use in daily practice.

### Continuing Education Credits

Psychologists and other healthcare providers may earn five continuing education credits for reading the books in the *Advances in Psychotherapy* series and taking a multiple-choice exam. This continuing education program is a partnership of Hogrefe Publishing and the National Register of Health Service Psychologists. Details are available at https://www.hogrefe.com/us/cenatreg

The National Register of Health Service Psychologists is approved by the American Psychological Association to sponsor continuing education for psychologists. The National Register maintains responsibility for this program and its content.

Advances in Psychotherapy – Evidence-Based Practice, Volume 51

# Occupational Stress

**Peter Y. Chen**

Department of Psychological Sciences, Auburn University, Auburn, AL

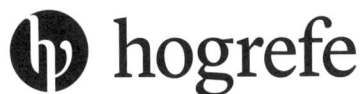

**Library of Congress of Congress Cataloging in Publication** information for the print version of this book is available via the Library of Congress Marc Database under the Library of Congress Control Number 2023937867

**Library and Archives Canada Cataloguing in Publication**

Title: Occupational stress / Peter Y. Chen, Department of Psychological Sciences, Auburn
  University, Auburn, AL.
Names: Chen, Peter Y., author.
Series: Advances in psychotherapy--evidence-based practice ; v. 51.
Description: Series statement: Advances in psychotherapy--evidence-based practice ; volume 51 |
  Includes bibliographical references.
Identifiers: Canadiana (print) 20230441394 | Canadiana (ebook) 20230441408 | ISBN 9780889375086
  (softcover) | ISBN 9781613345085 (EPUB) | ISBN 9781616765088 (PDF)
Subjects: LCSH: Job stress.
Classification: LCC HF5548.85 .C44 2023 | DDC 158.7/2—dc23

© 2024 by Hogrefe Publishing

www.hogrefe.com

PUBLISHING OFFICES

USA:        Hogrefe Publishing Corporation, 44 Merrimac St., Suite 207, Newburyport, MA 01950
            Phone 978 255 3700; E-mail customersupport@hogrefe.com

EUROPE:     Hogrefe Publishing GmbH, Merkelstr. 3, 37085 Göttingen, Germany
            Phone +49 551 99950 0, Fax +49 551 99950 111; E-mail publishing@hogrefe.com

SALES & DISTRIBUTION

USA:        Hogrefe Publishing, Customer Services Department,
            30 Amberwood Parkway, Ashland, OH 44805
            Phone 800 228 3749, Fax 419 281 6883; E-mail customersupport@hogrefe.com

UK:         Hogrefe Publishing, c/o Marston Book Services Ltd., 160 Eastern Ave.,
            Milton Park, Abingdon, OX14 4SB
            Phone +44 1235 465577, Fax +44 1235 465556; E-mail direct.orders@marston.co.uk

EUROPE:     Hogrefe Publishing, Merkelstr. 3, 37085 Göttingen, Germany
            Phone +49 551 99950 0, Fax +49 551 99950 111; E-mail publishing@hogrefe.com

OTHER OFFICES

CANADA:         Hogrefe Publishing Corporation, 82 Laird Drive, East York, Ontario, M4G 3V1

SWITZERLAND:    Hogrefe Publishing, Länggass-Strasse 76, 3012 Bern

Printed and bound in the USA

ISBN 978-0-88937-508-6 (print) · ISBN 978-1-61676-508-8 (PDF) · ISBN 978-1-61334-508-5 (EPUB)
https://doi.org/10.1027/00508-000

# Dedication

To my wife, Minehwa, for her unconditional support and love over 40 years.

To my son, Liwei, for his understanding and acceptance of who I am.

To my granddaughter, Marisol, for the joys she has brought to my life, and the time she spent with me while I was writing this book.

# Contents

# Preface

I started the journey of studying occupational stress when I was a graduate student. Immersed in theories, hypotheses, data analyses, and publications, I rarely spent time worrying about the employees behind each datapoint I collected ... until 1999.

Fast forward to 2007, Prof. Irvin Schonfeld asked me, as president of the Society for Occupational Health Psychology, to write an article in its inaugural newsletter. In the article, I reflected on what I had learned that day in 1999.

It was a colorful New England fall afternoon. A colleague stopped by my office and told me he had lost his job due to company-wide layoffs. He had worked at this company for about 20 years, and it had been his first job after he graduated from university. I walked with him in the company garden, and listened to him as he expressed frantic disbelief, anger, and fear. After approximately 30 minutes had passed, he told me his stomach was starting to ache badly. His physical and emotional pain struck me hard that day!

This incident and its impact, which I witnessed more than 2 decades ago, is one of the main reasons I decided to write this book that provides scientific reviews of the evidence regarding occupational stress, and which offers practical as well as evidence-based preventive management strategies to combat different job stressors (e.g., workplace misstatement, work–family conflict) that employees inevitably face daily.

Peter Y. Chen
May 2023
Auburn, Alabama

# 1

# Description

*No one should have to die while trying to make a living.*
Smallwood (2007)

Work provides employees with pride and a sense of purpose, and reinforces beliefs of being independent and resourceful. Yet, more than 60% of employed adults in 2019 identified work as a major source of stress in a survey conducted by the American Psychological Association (2019). It is not surprising that occupation stress has long been considered a national health problem by the US National Institute for Occupational Safety and Health (Sauter et al., 1990). This view has also been held by the International Labour Organization (ILO) (2016) and the European Agency for Safety and Health at Work (2018).

Because of the prevalence of stressful incidents encountered by people at work, the World Health Organization (WHO) (2019) recently included job stressors and their adverse outcomes in the 11th revision of the *International Statistical Classification of Diseases*. Similarly, a new diagnostic category of *trauma and stress-related disorders*, such as posttraumatic stress disorders resulting from encountering traumatic events at work (e.g., bullying), has been added into the 5th edition of the *Diagnostic and Statistical Manual of Mental Disorders* (American Psychiatric Association, 2013). Indeed, workplaces are constantly filled with psychosocial health hazards that paradoxically attenuate the expected benefits that the jobs could have offered.

A moral and ethical question is, how can our professionals put joint efforts into building a psychologically safe and healthy workplace for hardworking people around the world? Imagine an employee in Victoria, Australia, being constantly insulted and called ugly and fat by her coworkers. That was what 19-year-old waitress Brodie Panlock had experienced before she died by suicide (Brodie's Law, 2011). Also imagine the sanitation workers in Alabama who wore diapers to work because they were denied bathroom breaks outside of their sole 30-minute break per 8-hr shift (Southern Poverty Law Center, 2016). Imagine too, a female worker whose supervisor repeatedly made sexually explicit comments to her and other female coworkers. The supervisor also made lewd and vulgar gestures, and physically harassed his staff, for example, by pressing his private parts into one female worker's back. When she stood up to her supervisor, her hours were cut, she lost pay, and within a week she was fired (US EEOC v. New Breed Logistics, 2015). These cases may seem extreme, but similar cases continue to occur.

APA surveys from 2019 identified the workplace as a major source of stress

For instance, a series of workplace sexual harassment and assault cases have been revealed since the 2016 #MeToo movement, involving, for example, Roger Ailes at Fox News, Charlie Rose at PBS, Matt Lauer at NBC, the Royal Canadian Mounted Police, and the US Army. Recently, an executive at Imperial Pacific International (IPI) instructed a female employee to escort a drunk male customer to his villa, where she was forcefully kissed and subjected to unwelcome sexual propositions. IPI had a practice of retaliating against female employees for complaining about sexual harassment by terminating them or forcing them to quit (US Equal Employment Opportunity Commission, 2021).

Similarly, incidents of workplace aggression continue to occur. One afternoon in March 2021, an Uber driver in San Francisco, Subhakar Khadka, was cursed, attacked, coughed on, and pepper-sprayed by two female passengers. And just for a moment, pretend you're Amazon warehouse worker, Jenny. She leaves her post for a 30-minute lunch break, and the clock starts counting down immediately. Jenny needs to walk across a warehouse the size of 14 football fields to access the cafeteria for a $4 cold sandwich. If she makes it within 30 minutes, she is lucky. If she does not, she may suffer adverse consequences, including a pay cut or even job loss (Associated Press, 2021).

A recent report revealed that Japan's extreme overwork culture (working long hours, working more days, and not taking holiday leave) persists, even after the first case of *karoshi* (overwork death) was reported in 1969, and the Work Style Reform Bill was passed to address overwork issues in 2018. A Japanese engineer, Hideyuki, with two children aged 4 and 6 years, took only 2 days off from work in 2019, which was more than in previous years, even though he is entitled to 20 days annual leave. He was too afraid of his manager saying something for taking days off (BBC, 2020).

Occupational stress research over the past century has provided convincing evidence that stressful working conditions likely adversely affect workers' immune systems, physical and mental health, and the well-being of their families. In addition, stressful work conditions are associated with disruption to organizational growth and societal progress (Chen et al., 2023). Hassard et al. (2018a) estimated the economic cost resulting from stressful job experience in eight developed countries: It ranged from US $221.13 million to US $187 billion per year, of which productivity loss accounted for 70% to 90% and health care costs accounted for 10% to 30%. Furthermore, the WHO and the ILO have jointly estimated that 488 million people, or 8.9% of the global population, worked more than 55 hrs per week in 2016 (Descatha et al., 2021). In addition, Descatha et al. (2021) have estimated that 745,194 deaths and 23.3 million disability-adjusted life years from ischemic heart disease and stroke combined were attributable to overwork.

Is making a living worth the risk of a worker's well-being? It is the central question we shall contemplate throughout this book. I will first provide a description of key concepts, including occupations, occupational stress, job stressors, and consequences of job stressors in Chapter 1. In Chapter 2, I will discuss how work conditions and organizational characteristics pose threats or harms to people's well-being and how organizational improvements can be made, via the lens of prominent occupation stress theories or models, including role stress theory, transactional theory, person–environment fit theory, and the job demands–resources theory (including the effort–reward imbalance model, the demands–control model, and the demands–control-support model). These theoretical frameworks shed light on how exposure to job stressors adversely affect people's well-being and the growth of an organization. Furthermore, these frameworks provide directions for how to proactively combat and manage job stressors and job strains.

In Chapter 3, I introduce the major job stressors identified by Burke (2019), Goh et al. (2015), the ILO (2016), McGrath (1976), and Sonnentag and Frese (2003). These frequently encountered job stressors include role stressors (role conflict, role ambiguity, role overload, and illegitimate tasks), work versus family and nonwork conflict, workload and workplace telepressure, lack of control or autonomy, organizational constraints, organizational justice, organizational politics, and workplace mistreatment. Adverse impacts of these job stressors are also presented primarily based on meta-analytic results when available.

Finally, in Chapter 4, I will describe organizational stress management intervention programs which are preventive in nature. These intervention programs are designed to help employees recover from work (Hahn et al., 2011); to craft employees' job demands and resources via seeking resources, seeking challenges, and optimizing job demands (Demerouti et al., 2020); to promote supervisory support to reduce work-family conflict (Odle-Dusseau et al., 2016); to promote supervisory support to prevent abusive and uncivil behaviors (Gonzalez-Morales et al., 2018), and to redesign work to promote job control (Bond & Bunce, 2001; Holman & Axtell, 2016; Logan & Ganster, 2005).

## 1.1    Terminology and Definitions

### 1.1.1    Occupations

To better understand occupational stress, it is helpful to know first what an occupation entails, as well as the relationship between an occupation and people who work in that occupation. As an example, I will use information provided by the Occupational Information Network (O*NET) (2021) to explain what the occupation of, for example, "a mental health counselor" entails. That refers to *a collection of similar job titles* such as mental health specialist, mental health therapist, behavior analyst, or correctional counselor. In general, a group of people with similar job titles engages in certain prescribed tasks or work activities to achieve organizational goals. Work activities for mental health counselors may include counseling clients regarding their personal needs, or teaching clients life skills or coping strategies. These activities are often performed in face-to-face discussions with others, often working indoors and using email, and mental health counselors have quite

> Occupational Information Network database of approx. 1,000 occupations (US Employment and Training Administration)

a lot of freedom to make decisions without supervision. To perform these work activities, mental health counselors are required to be knowledgeable (e.g., knowledge of principles, methods, and procedures for diagnosis, treatment, and rehabilitation of physical and mental dysfunctions, and for career counseling and guidance), have certain skills (e.g., be aware of others' reactions and understand why they react as they do), abilities (e.g., to listen to and understand information and ideas presented through spoken words and sentences), job experience (e.g., the job requires extensive experience), and education (e.g., most counselors have an advanced degree).

Work activities in any occupation, as well as required knowledge, skills, abilities, and other characteristics to perform work activities, play an import role in any understanding of occupational stress, and that includes the contexts in which the work activities are performed. There are various social and physical factors associated with those work contexts, which influence how people do their work. People in some occupations may be inherently exposed to higher risks of occupation-related physical and mental health than people in other occupations. For instance, drywall installers use their hands and arms to install big, heavy drywalls onto vertical or horizontal surfaces repetitively each day. Because their work contexts consist of physical demands, drywall installers in this occupation are at a higher risk of suffering musculoskeletal injuries or disorders in their back and shoulder areas, such as rotator cuff tendonitis or tendon strain (Chiou et al., 2000). Similarly, police patrol officers maintain order and protect life while they are exposed to life-threatening or emotionally draining events during their shift. For example, they regularly have to handle abused children or domestic violence, encounter people who have been killed or injured, or assist people in distress. The physical and social demands inherent in these work contexts put first responders at a higher risk of physical and mental illness, such as cardiovascular disease (CVD) morbidity or burnout (Zimmerman, 2012).

In addition to the physical and social factors associated with work contexts, which influence how people do things, organizational characteristics affect people's behaviors and attitudes. Imagine people in the same occupation but working in two different organizations: organization A and B. In organization A, uncivil and abusive behaviors are not disciplined or penalized, interpersonal conflict occurs frequently, and productivity and profits are valued more than employees' health and safety. Organization B is the opposite of organization A. It does not take a rocket scientist to predict that people from the two organizations would have very different work experiences, emotions, attitudes, and interaction relationships, as well as ways of doing their work, even for people who hold the same or similar job titles.

## 1.1.2   Occupational Stress

Over the past century, we have witnessed an increase in occupational stress research. In a centennial special issue of the *Journal of Applied Psychology*, Bliese et al. (2017) tallied up an increase of occupational stress research from 173 articles (1917–1966), to 213 articles (1967–1996), to 220 articles (1997–2017). Since *Work & Stress,* a journal specifically devoted to occupational stress research, was first published in 1987, other journals with similar scopes have emerged, including *Journal of Occupational Health Psychology* (first published in 1997), *International Journal of Stress Management* (in 2003), and *Occupational Health Science* (in 2017).

While there are many journals devoted to occupational stress research, the term "occupational stress," has been interpreted differently by different people, including researchers. First, occupational stress has been referred to as work-related stimuli or job stressors posing a threat to workers' well-being or behaviors. *Job stressors* can be any work-related stressful event, such as being yelled at by a boss or receiving conflicting or incorrect instructions from supervisors while performing a task. Job stressors can also be characteristics of a job, such as the fast pace of cutting in a meat-packing facility, little freedom to make decisions, or a 12-hr shift in a remote area each day for a few continuous weeks followed by several days off at home.

Yet occupational stress has also been referred to as *job strain* or the individual response to job stressors. This view is rooted in an early view of stress as a *fight or flight* reaction. In sum, occupational stress is often interpreted as (1) job stressors (i.e., work-related stressful events or the characteristics of a job), (2) job strains (i.e., employees' responses to job stressors), or (3) both job strains and job stressors (Jex et al., 1992).

To avoid confusion when using the word "stress," I specifically refer to job stressors as stressful events at work or job characteristics, and job strains as employees' reactions to perceived stressful events. Furthermore, I refer to occupational stress as a body of research (McGrath, 1976) or as a process: "A situation wherein job-related factors interact with a worker to change (i.e., disrupt or enhance) his or her psychological and/or physiological condition such that the person (i.e., mind-body) is forced to deviate from normal functioning" (Beehr & Newman, 1978, p. 669–670).

**Job stressors vs. job strains**

The effects of job stressors on workers have generally been studied in field settings. Without an adequate research design, such as manipulating job stressors in a controlled setting, it is challenging for occupational stress researchers to provide definitive evidence for causal effects in field research. Two classic stress studies, however, have provided convincing evidence regarding the negative impacts of stressful events. The first study showed that stressful life events increased the rate of infection among healthy people who reported major stressful life events (Cohen et al., 1991). Healthy subjects in this study received one of five respiratory viruses or saline (placebo) via nasal drops. They also reported the number of major life events that had had negative impacts on them in the past year, their ability to cope with current demands, and negative emotions. These measures subsequently formed a psychological stress index via a principal component analysis. The research team found that an increase in psychological stress index was associated with an increase in infection rate after controlling for more than 15 potential confounding variables (e.g., personality variables, health practices, white cell counts prior to being exposed).

The second study showed that an increase of daily stressful events was related to a smaller number of antibodies found in saliva (Stone et al., 1994). Middle-aged men in the study reviewed 80 events that had occurred in the past 24 hrs for up to 12 weeks. Each event was rated daily on a scale from extremely desirable to extremely undesirable. Results showed that an increase in desirable events was positively associated with an increase in antibodies. In contrast, there is a negative relationship between the number of undesirable events and antibodies. Interestingly, while the research team investigated events classified by content (e.g., work, leisure, household), they found a negative relationship between undesirable events at work and antibodies, but there was no relationship between desirable events at work and antibodies. Overall, both studies provide convincing causal evidence that stressful events likely adversely affect our well-being.

### 1.1.3    Job Stressors

Work conditions play a vital role in shaping people's perceptions. Yet, the same work condition (e.g., being given a lot of responsibilities to organize workflows) may be perceived as stressful by one individual but not by another. Therefore, it is important to recognize the important role of personal appraisal, perception, and/or interpretation of work conditions, and distinguish between work conditions and perceived work conditions, while studying job stressors, defined as work conditions *appraised* to be stressful, threatening, or harmful. It is *perceived* stressful work conditions (being appraised as such) that I will focus on in this book.

#### Chronic and Acute Job Stressors

Job stressors can be classified into two categories based on the duration and frequency of stressful events: *chronic job stressors* and *acute job stressors*. Chronic job stressors can further be classified as *chronic intermittent job stressors* and *chronic prolonged job stressors* (Chen, 1991). Chronic intermittent job stressors occur periodically – for example, having a weekly meeting with a rude colleague. In contrast, chronic prolonged job stressors persist continuously for a long period of time, such as having an abusive supervisor who often yells at their subordinates.

There are two types of acute job stressors: *acute time-limited job stressors* and *acute sequential job stressors* (Chen, 1991). Acute time-limited job stressors appear during a very short period, such as during an explosion in a factory, or the temporary closure of a restaurant due to a natural disaster. Acute sequential job stressors emerge over an extended period as the result of initial events. For example, using the example of an explosion in a factory, employees may need to work at unusually high speeds to make up for production losses, or with regard to a restaurant closure, the business may face unexpected financial challenges.

## Challenge and Hindrance Stressors

Some conventionally studied stressful events (e.g., working under tight deadlines) have been found to be either *positively correlated* or *uncorrelated* with job satisfaction and performance (e.g., Payne et al., 1988). These patterns have led researchers to classify job stressors a priori into either challenge or hindrance stressors. *Challenge stressors* may lead to strain yet energize people to accomplish tasks at the same time. In contrast, *hindrance stressors* lead to strain without energizing people (Horan et al., 2020). However, as Horan et al. pointed out, both types of job stressor are not mutually exclusive, solely appraised by people, and not static across different time, circumstances, and occupations. Simply put, the same work conditions (e.g., challenging projects) or job characteristics (e.g., responsibilities to make consequential decisions) may or may not be appraised as stressful by different people at different times, under different circumstances, or holding different occupations. As shown by Webster et al. (2011), people appraise the same job stressors as both challenges and hindrances to varying degrees.

## Regulation Uncertainty, Regulation Obstacles, and Overtaxing Regulations

Another way to categorize job stressors is based on types of disruption or disturbance in the process of regulating people's actions to perform work activities or achieve expected goals (Frese & Zapf, 1994). People are generally motivated to pursue goals to meet their needs. These goals can be to become rich, to obtain a medical degree, to read a book, to learn a foreign language, to find a spouse, etc. While pursuing goals at work, we constantly regulate our actions (e.g., using tools or technologies, planning a sequence of work activities, modifying plans, coordinating activities or other plans, involving other team members, developing new tasks or new plans). Emphasis on how action regulations are disturbed or disrupted offers insightful understanding about job stressors because the same work conditions or job characteristics may or may not be perceived as stressful within-person and/or between-persons across time. This classification also explains why a work condition, or a job characteristic may affect our regulations via more than one type of disruption. In other words, a job stressor can be categorized by more than one type of disruption. Because of its flexibility and explanatory utility, in this book, this classification is chosen to explain how key job stressors affect people at work.

According to Frese and Zapf (1994), there are three types of regulation disruption: *regulation uncertainty*, *regulation obstacles*, and *overtaxing regulations*. Regulation uncertainty occurs when people are unsure how to accomplish assignments or work activities, because of too much work or a lack of needed knowledge, skills and abilities, or other experience. It could also happen when individuals are uncertain or unable to assess which courses of action should be taken to achieve goals. Furthermore, individuals may experience uncertainty about their actions when they receive insufficient or delayed feedback from others (Jackson & Schuler, 1985). Other examples include situations in which individuals are unclear about their duties, roles, or the expectations on them, or when individuals receive two or more conflicting instructions or expectations. Overall, these uncertain conditions are stressful because employees' regulation of actions are disrupted, which interferes with their ability to achieve their goals.

The second type of disruption is regulation obstacles, which refers to objects or conditions that interfere with people's ability to perform work activities and disrupt actions that help them achieve their goals. It can be extremely frustrating when people do not have the needed tools, equipment, materials, supplies, budgetary support, job-related authority, or other resources to perform their work activities (Peters et al., 1980). This can also happen when people's actions are disrupted by other people or external conditions. Imagine the anxiety and fear that poultry workers experienced when they did not have adequate personal protection equipment and could not maintain social distances at work during the COVID-19 pandemic! Similarly, working parents, particularly women, experience tremendous conflicting pressures while juggling work and family (either work interferes with family, or family interferes with work; Carlson et al., 2000). Often, regulation obstacles can be colleagues or supervisors with whom people work. For instance, people may feel threatened and hurt at work if their coworkers often shut them out of the conversation or ridicule their opinions or appearance, or supervisors keep important work-related information from them (Howard et al., 2020).

Overtaxing regulation, the third type of disruption, refers to the speed and intensity of regulating people's action to accomplish goals. People often experience pressures and exert high energy at the same time to get tasks done under time constraints, even if they have the needed knowledge, skills, abilities, etc. Yet, work conditions or certain job characteristics with a persistent requirement to be fast paced and use intensive energy can disrupt how people regulate their actions to achieve competing goals, because their mental and physical capabilities may gradually become worn out. Imagine working parents constantly juggling their time among taking care of their children, maintaining their marital relationship, pursuing individual interests and hobbies, completing dynamic and challenging tasks, and working with people with different interests or ideas. Their actions to achieve multiple goals are inevitably disrupted by demands from different sources.

## 1.1.4   Causal Relations: Job Stressors and Strains

Most occupational stress research has been conducted via cross-sectional designs, which limit any causal conclusions that can be made about adverse effects of job stressors on job strains. Evidence documenting the adverse effects of stressors on strains has been demonstrated with rigorous research design (e.g., Cohen et al., 1991; Stone et al., 1994). Contrary to the conventional wisdom, however, strains (e.g., burnout) or individual characteristics (e.g., anxiety) may also create stressors in some circumstances.

Spector et al. (2000) proposed the stressor creation hypothesis in which people with certain dispositions, such as high levels of neuroticism or depression, may get into conflicts with others more often and manage work activities less efficiently. In addition, their neurotic or depressed behaviors likely instigate negative reactions from others at work, which in turn make them feel more anxious or depressed. Furthermore, jobs with certain characteristics attract employees with certain characteristics. Spector et al. (1995) have documented that people with high levels of anxiety tend to be found in jobs with low job autonomy (a job stressor to be discussed in Chapter 3), and people with high levels of optimism tend to be found in jobs with high job autonomy.

Bakker and Demerouti (2017) have also provided evidence to support the proposition that job strains likely create job stressors. People with high levels of job strain tend to create obstacles by themselves and self-undermine regulation of their actions. As a result of job strains, these self-undermining behaviors (e.g., poor skills in communication and emotional control, low job performance, and poor interpersonal relationships) subsequently create more job stressors as well as cyclical job strains over time.

Furthermore, reciprocal effects between job stressors and job strains have been demonstrated in a recent meta-analysis. Based on 48 longitudinal studies, Guthier et al. (2020) found evidence that job stressors and burnout were reciprocally associated. Foremost, the size of the effect of job stressors on burnout (i.e., stressor effect) over time tended to be smaller than that of burnout on job stressors (i.e., strain effect) over time. In sum, the above review suggests that job stressors and job strains could be reciprocally related if examined over time. Under either stressor-effect or strain-effect circumstances over time, employees' regulations of work activities are nonetheless disrupted. In the next section, we will survey what consequences of job stressors have been studied in occupational stress research.

**There is evidence for a reciprocal relationship between job stressors and job strains over time**

## 1.1.5    Consequences of Job Stressors

Variables used to study the consequences of job stressors are typically classified into four levels: *process*, *individual and family*, *organizational*, and *societal/national* (Beehr & Newman, 1978; Hassard et al., 2018a). I will present the consequences of each level in the following sections. References regarding self-reports of widely studied individual and family level outcome variables are listed in Appendix 1.

### Process Level Variables
This group consists of variables that are considered to be intermediate or mediating variables that link between actual job stressors and individual outcomes. Neurological reactions, physiological arousals, emotions, perception of the environment, appraisal or interpretation of the environment, and decisions to respond or not, as well as other cognitive processes such as working memory, executive function, and self-regulation (Beehr & Newman, 1978;

Rafaeli et al., 2012) are examples of process variables within individuals. Because process variables occur within individuals, these variables are inevitably influenced by individual characteristics and dispositions such as self-efficacy, self-esteem, optimism, the Big Five personality traits (i.e., Openness, Conscientiousness, Extraversion, Neuroticism, and Agreeableness), locus of control, workaholism, Type A behavior patterns, and hardiness. Discussion of individual characteristics and dispositions, however, is beyond the scope of this book.

### Individual and Family Level Variables

Consequences of job stressors at this level include four main categories of outcomes: physical, psychological, behavioral, and family. Although these outcomes are described separately in each of the sections that follow, inter-relationships among these categories should be underscored. For instance, obesity (a physical outcome) is often related to overeating or alcohol use (behavioral outcomes).

#### *Physical Outcomes*

Physical outcomes generally include cardiovascular problems (heart rate, blood pressure), ischemic heart disease, stroke, biochemical problems (abnormal levels of uric acid, blood sugar, steroid hormones such as cortisol, cholesterol, catecholamines), immune system problems, gastrointestinal problems such as peptic ulcers, inflammation problems, psychosomatic problems (e.g., sleep disturbance), musculoskeletal problems, obesity, suicide, and mortality (Chen et al., 2023; Ganster et al., 2018; Goh et al., 2016).

#### *Psychological Outcomes*

Psychological outcomes, either self-reported or reported by others, include job satisfaction, health satisfaction, life satisfaction, well-being, boredom, fatigue, frustration, moodiness, anger, anxiety, depression, detachment from work, rumination, job involvement, hostility, organizational commitment (consisting of *affective commitment*, which is emotional attachment to an organization, *continuance commitment*, which is attachment to an organization because of an inability to quit, and *normative commitment*, which is attachment to an organization because of feeling obligated to stay; Allen & Meyer, 1996). Other outcomes include burnout (consisting of *emotional exhaustion*, which is feeling unable to devote more to a job emotionally, *cynicism* which is distancing from one's work, colleagues, or clients and becoming cynical about others, and *reduced personal accomplishment*, which is experiencing a sense of professional incompetence; Maslach et al., 2001) and *reduced job engagement* (i.e., low energy and effort toward job and organization; Schaufeli et al., 2002).

#### *Behavioral Outcomes*

Behavioral outcomes include unhealthy behaviors (alcohol and drug abuse, smoking, overeating), emotion regulations and control, decision errors, poor job or task performance, behaviors that harm organizations or people at work (e.g., antisocial behaviors, aggressive behaviors, deviant behaviors, counterproductive work behaviors, uncivil behaviors, abusive supervision, etc.), accidents, injuries, discretionary behaviors that benefit other individuals (or organizational citizenship behavior targeted at individuals), discretionary behaviors that benefit organizations (i.e., organizational citizenship behavior targeted at an organization), absenteeism, lateness, going to work sick (i.e., presenteeism), turnover intention, and turnover. Spector (1998) considered some of the behavioral outcomes as individual coping responses that either reduce emotional responses (emotion-focused) or address job stressors directly or indirectly (problem-focused). Prevention programs designed to reduce emotional responses (e.g., recovery training or job crafting training), prevent job stressors (e.g., job crafting training or supportive supervisor training), or redesign stressful job characteristics (e.g., work design) will be described in detail in Chapter 4.

### *Family Outcomes*

Family outcomes include children's health, problem behaviors, and physical activity; family function (performance) and satisfaction; parenting behaviors and satisfaction; quality of family life; marital adjustment, satisfaction, and related stress; family-related strain; or satisfaction with leisure activities. Prevention programs that specifically reduce work–family conflict by increasing family supportive supervisor behaviors will be illustrated in Chapter 4.

## Organizational Level Variables

Outcomes associated with job stressors at this level may include profit; productivity; costs associated with turnover, absenteeism, and presenteeism; costs associated with health care and insurance premiums; costs associated with workers' compensation and insurance premiums, disability claims, litigations and associated costs, deaths, strikes, or reputational damage. Relatively few studies have been conducted in the occupational stress literature on organizational level variables – with a few exceptions (e.g., Ganster et al., 2001; Grinza & Rycx, 2020; Schmidt et al., 2019).

## Societal and National Level Variables

The impacts of job stressors at the societal and national level are often gauged by direct or indirect costs of national productivity loss (sickness absenteeism, presenteeism), tax revenue loss, and medical claims or health care expenditures that are attributed to job stressors. In addition, these impacts can be measured by mortality and morbidity. Finally, some impacts can be inferred from the legislation established in countries that address a particular job stressor such as age discrimination, racial discrimination, gender discrimination, sexual harassment, workplace bullying, or overwork death (Chen et al., 2023). Similar to the situation for organizational level variables, fewer studies have been conducted to examine the societal/national impacts of specific or general job stressors – with a few exceptions (e.g., Goh et al., 2015; Goh et al., 2016; Hassard et al., 2018a, 2018b; Hassard et al., 2019).

# 2

# Theories and Models

What work conditions and organizational characteristics pose threats to or harm people's well-being? How are these conditions and characteristics perceived or appraised to be stressful? How does exposure to these conditions and characteristics adversely affect people's well-being and organizational growth? To what extent are these adverse effects attributed to work conditions and organizational characteristics, people, or interactions between situations and people? What are the scientific approaches that can reduce or amend these conditions and characteristics, or minimize the adverse effects of these conditions and characteristics? These are just a few very important questions that are explored in Chapters 3 and 4 via the lens of major occupational stress theories, including role stress theory (Kahn et al., 1964), transactional theory (Lazarus & Folkman, 1987), person–environment fit (PE fit) theory (Caplan, 1987), the effort–reward imbalance model (Siegrist, 1996), the demands–control model (Karasek, 1979), the demands–control–support model (Johnson & Hall, 1988), and the job demands–resources (JD-R) theory (Demerouti et al., 2001).

## 2.1 Role Stress Theory

**Role stressors occur when role-related activities are disrupted**

Employees hold a variety of roles where they are expected to fulfill formal job responsibilities and duties. For instance, a human resources specialist plays the role of recruiting job applicants, selecting qualified job applicants, hiring employees, maintaining and processing paperwork (e.g., hiring, termination, retirement, transfer, promotions), addressing employee relation issues (e.g., harassment complaints), or maintaining current knowledge of employment guidelines and laws. They may also be expected to play a nonprescribed role such as helping a newcomer, being a good organizational citizen, being a hard worker, maintaining strong social networks, and so on. In addition, they have other expected roles outside of the work domain, such as being a daughter, a wife, a mother, a volunteer, a friend, a political party member, or a community member, etc. These multiple roles become the core of our identities, and partially shape our values, attitudes, beliefs, and behaviors. The more diverse our roles and the more tasks that are assigned to us, the more our identities are formulated, and the greater the difficulty in being able to juggle the responsibilities of numerous roles at the same time (Stryker &

Burke, 2000). *Role stress theory* (Kahn et al., 1964) suggests that our actions to achieve role-related activities can be disrupted or disturbed when there are conflicting or incompatible expectations of roles, ambiguous expectations of roles, or overtaxing expectations of roles. Role-related job stressors such as role conflict, role ambiguity, illegitimate tasks, role overload, and work–family conflict will be discussed in Chapter 3.

## 2.2 Transactional Theory

Job stressors are classified based on three types of disruption or disturbance in the process of regulating people's actions to perform work activities or achieving expected goals (Frese & Zapf, 1994). Yet not all people would appraise the same events as disruptive or stressful, and not all people would cope with stressful events similarly. As Lazarus and Folkman (1987) suggested, we cannot understand emotional responses toward these events and experiences solely from a person or environment perspective. Instead, emotional reactions toward stressful experiences occur when a person interacts with the environment.

According to the transactional theory of Lazarus and Folkman (1987), there are two major processes – *cognitive appraisal* and *coping* – involved in the transaction in the stressful person–environment relationship. The first process, cognitive appraisal, occurs when an employee evaluates whether a work condition poses any harm, threat, or challenge to their well-being and how the condition affects them – these are referred to as the *primary appraisal*. If the condition is evaluated as harmful, threatening, or challenging to their well-being, what can they do (i.e., what are their coping options) under these circumstances – referred to as their *secondary appraisal*.

**Employees engage in cognitive appraisal to evaluate a work condition**

In the context of occupational stress, employees engage in the primary appraisal to evaluate how they are affected by an encounter. For example, they may lose self-respect when an abusive supervisor yells at them, or aspirations to excel at work may decrease when their opinions at team meetings are often ignored, or they may not be able to accomplish an important project by the deadline because they do not have sufficient resources.

In secondary appraisals, employees assess coping options regarding to what extent the situation they encounter could be changed, must be accepted, could be acted on after gathering more information, or require them to hold back from doing what they want to do (Folkman et al., 1986). Lazarus and Folkman (1987) further considered these options – the extent to which situations could be changed (i.e., changeability) and situations that must be accepted (i.e., controllability) – as more useful from theoretical and empirical viewpoints than other coping options.

The second process, coping, refers to constant changes in cognitive or behavioral efforts to manage external and/or internal demands that overtax one's resources. Specifically, coping arises from cognitive appraisals of harm, threat, or challenges from encountered demands and available resources to

**Coping is an effort to manage external and/or internal demands**

manage these demands. The coping process constantly changes across time and situations (Lazarus & Folkman, 1987; Folkman et al., 1986).

There are two major functions of coping: *regulating stressful emotions* (i.e., emotion-focused coping) and *modifying stressful person–environment relationships* that cause strains (i.e., problem-focused coping). The majority of people use both functions when experiencing stressful events. Further, Lazarus and Folkman (1987) showed that problem-focused forms of coping (e.g., seeking support from supervisors, modifying work processes) tend to be in response to contextual factors, yet some forms of emotion-focused coping tend to be stable and may be influenced by person factors. Because cognitive and behavioral efforts change constantly, Folkman et al. (1986) do not make an a priori assumption about what constitutes effective (or good) or ineffective (or bad) coping, which is simply defined as a person's effort to manage stressful events. Indeed, the favorable or unfavorable results of any given coping process are contingent upon (1) who uses it, (2) when it is used, (3) under what circumstances, and (4) which types of criteria are chosen to evaluate that result (Lazarus & Folkman, 1987).

Latack (1986) further showed that both functions can be seen as either taking charge of a situation (e.g., get together with my supervisor to discuss the problem I face, or think about the challenges I can identify in this situation in order to regulate my emotions) or avoiding a situation (e.g., avoid being in certain situations to reduce stressful encounters, or remind myself that work is not everything, so that I can regulate my emotions).

It should also be noted that there are other conceptual coping responses beyond these two functions of coping. For instance, Latack (1986) added a third category, *symptom management*, to manage symptoms related to job stressors, rather than to manage threatening stressors themselves. These strategies may include getting extra sleep, taking time off from work, daydreaming, or watching TV. Similarly, Carver et al. (1989) include three *less useful* coping responses (venting emotions, behavioral disengagement, and mental disengagement), which are not considered either problem-focused coping or emotional-focused coping.

In contrast to role stress theory, transaction theory does not specifically identify what encounters or situations are considered as job stressors. Instead, it highlights the roles of cognitive appraisal and coping process in the transaction between an employee and a work environment. A high job demand may be mitigated by effective coping efforts or behaviors, yet a low job demand may leave an employee vulnerable if they do not have the skills or abilities to cope effectively with it. Several preventive measures to combat job demands and their impacts at work and off work will be described in Chapter 4.

## 2.3    Person–Environment Fit Theory

There are many person–environment fit (PE fit) theories applied to investigate multidisciplinary topics such as job satisfaction, quality of life, work adjustment, vocational choice, socialization, recruitment–selection–retention, work design, or occupational stress (van Vianen, 2018). In the context of occupational stress, PE fit refers to the goodness of fit, correspondence, or compatibility between personal attributes (e.g., needs, goals, values, skills, abilities) and environmental attributes (e.g., supplies, demands, job characteristics). Similar to transaction theory (Lazarus & Folkman, 1987), PE fit theory considers person–environment relations, and implicitly assumes that the environment is cognitively appraised by the person.

Occupational stress research has generally focused on two types of PE fit (Caplan, 1987; Edwards & Cooper, 1990): the compatibility between environmental *supplies* and personal *values* (i.e., SV fit), and the compatibility between environmental *demands* and personal *abilities* (DA fit). *SV fit* refers to the extent to which employees' needs, motives, desires, preferences, and goals are fulfilled by supplies provided by their jobs, or employees' desires are met by what they actually receive from their jobs. SV misfit becomes a source of job strains when an employee's desires, needs, motives, preferences, or goals are not met with those provided by his or her job. *DA fit* focuses on the extent to which employees' knowledge, skills, and abilities correspond with what their jobs require, or whether environmental demands exceed employees' abilities and skills. DA misfit becomes a source of job strains when job requirements do not correspond with an employee's knowledge, abilities, and/or skills. There are other types of PE fit that are also relevant to occupational stress, such as person–team fit that focuses on interpersonal compatibility between a team member and their work team, or person–supervisor fit that focuses on the compatibility of the dyadic relationship between an employee and their supervisor (Kristof-Brown et al., 2005).

A misfit or incompatibility, regardless of its direction (van Vianen, 2018), between person and supervisor, person and team, or person and job (i.e., supplies–values and demands–abilities), inevitably disrupts action regulations (Frese & Zapf, 1994). Regulation uncertainty occurs, for example, when employees are uncertain about whether their tasks are on track, because they rarely receive timely feedback from their supervisor or team members, or when employees are uncertain if their hard work is being recognized or rewarded (see Section 1.1.3). Regulation obstacles, on the other hand, occur when the required resources are not supplied and employees are not able to perform their tasks, or when incompatible relationships among members lead to a stalled team (see Section 1.1.3). Overtaxing regulations occur when, for example, employees experience a high workload or have a poor relationship with their supervisor, which in turn overtax their abilities or capabilities to perform work activities well (see Section 1.1.3).

Edwards and Cooper (1990) articulate the concept of fit from three different perspectives. The first form of fit focuses on the discrepancy between personal attributes (P) and work environment (E), and the discrepancy form of fit is associated with increased job strains. The second form of fit focuses on the interaction between P and E, and the interaction form of fit indicates that the relationship between the attributes of the E and job strain is contingent upon P. The third form focuses on the proportion of P that is met by E, and the proportion form indicates that P serves as a standard by which E is compared (it is a characteristic of discrepancy form), and P influences the relationship between E and job strain (it is a characteristic of interaction form). Furthermore, the proportion form suggests that the relationship between E and job strain diminishes when P increases (e.g., an improvement in an individual's skills or social relationships). Overall, preventive interventions can aim at changing P (e.g., reframing preferences, improving skills, seeking job resources and challenges, or minimizing demands), modifying E (e.g., providing needed resources, reducing job demands, or redesigning job or organizational characteristics), and altering a combination of P and E.

Kristof-Brown et al. (2005) meta-analyzed the relationships of DA fit, SV fit, person-team fit, and person-supervisor fit with stress-related outcomes. Overall, perceived fits were associated with increased job satisfaction, commitment to organization, and satisfaction with coworker or supervisor. Person-team fit and person-supervisor fit were positively associated with job performance.

## 2.4   Job Demands–Resources Theory

Over the past 20 years, the job demands–resources (JD-R) theory (Bakker & Demerouti, 2014, 2017; Demerouti et al., 2001) has become a popular occupational stress theory, which has been widely examined and meta-analyzed in areas of occupational health (Crawford et al., 2010) and safety (see a meta-analysis by Nahrgang et al., 2011). Bakker and Demerouti (2014) stated that the JD-R theory they developed was inspired by the effort–reward imbalance model (Siegrist, 1996), demands–control model (Karasek, 1979), and demands–control–support model (Johnson & Hall, 1988). To provide an adequate background for JD-R theory, each of these models will first be described.

### 2.4.1   Effort–Reward Imbalance Model

**Imbalance between the rewards and efforts can be a source of job strains**

Siegrist (1996) proposed the effort–reward imbalance model, which explains the emotional distress, autonomic arousal, and physical strains resulting from the imbalance between a high effort a person devotes to their work and the lower-than-expected reward they receive. This imbalance condition deviates from expected reciprocity and norms of social exchanges. The model is similar to the PE fit theory; however, the misfit or incongruence of this model focuses solely on the relationship between *rewards* (money, esteem and approval, and status control) and *efforts*, including those of the latter that are attributed to extrinsic sources such as job demands (workload or work pressure) and obligations, or to intrinsic sources such as an employee's motivation or need for control in a demanding situation.

High effort and low reward conditions are considered high cost and low gain situations – situations that people prefer to avoid. Yet Siegrist (1996) pointed out that people often engage in unfavorable trade-offs, especially those with few job options, and particularly those with low levels of occupational status control, including forced mobility, few promotion prospects, job insecurity, or status inconsistency. After all, the cost of being demoted, terminated, or unemployed outweighs the cost of exerting high efforts for inadequate rewards. When people chronically exert high efforts yet receive low rewards at work, they are at a higher risk of experiencing negative emotions and recurrent autonomic activation, which strains cardiovascular and hormonal systems in the long run. Siegrist reported an association between an imbalance condition and increased hypertension, higher levels of low-density lipoprotein (LDL) cholesterol, acute myocardial infarctions, coronary heart disease, stroke, or sudden cardiac death among blue collar workers. Thus far, positive associations between imbalance (operationalized by the interaction between effort and reward) and CVD mortality and morbidity have been reported in eight studies, six of which utilized a prospective design, based on a review by van Vegchel et al. (2005). van Vegchel et al. further showed that the imbalance condition had been reported to be associated with CVD symptoms and/or risk factors (e.g., hypertension and cholesterol) in 13 out of 15 studies, and with poor job-related well-being (e.g., burnout and job satisfaction) in five out of six studies.

### 2.4.2  Demands–Control Model

Karasek (1979) proposed an influential occupational stress model, the demands–control model, that broadly impacts multiple disciplines, including occupational medicine, nursing, industrial engineering, human factors, sociology, epidemiology, and psychology (Luchman & González-Morales, 2013; van der Doef & Maes, 1999). The demands–control model, a stress-management model applied for work design, postulates that mental strains result from a joint effect (i.e., interaction) of job demands and job decision latitude or job control.

Although both job demands and job decision latitude are not clearly defined by Karasek, one can infer the definitions based on the measures used in his study. Essentially, *job demands* are job characteristics that either require employees to work fast or hard, or carry out a great deal of work often under tight deadlines, or they consist of conflicting demands from others. *Job decision latitude*, a term often used interchangeably with *job control*, discretion, or freedom to make a decision, refers to *skill discretion, decision authority,* or both. A job with a high level of skill discretion requires employees to engage in work activities with high skill levels, and employees in these positions are required to learn new things. In addition, this job characteristic offers

**Job control refers to an employee's discretion whether, when, or how to engage in work activities**

opportunities for employees to engage in nonrepetitive work activities, and requires them to be creative at work. A job with a high level of decision authority means that employees have freedom in how to work, can make a lot of decisions, or they have a say over what happens (Karasek, 1979).

When employees experience high levels of job demands and decision latitudes simultaneously, they need to engage in many problem-solving activities with a high level of responsibility. As a result, they likely gain brand new knowledge and develop additional skills either on or off the job. According to the *strain hypothesis* (Karasek, 1979), under a high level of job demands, however, employees tend to suffer mental strains if they have little or inadequate decision latitude to make a decision, due to an organization's authority structure, bureaucratic norms, technology, or other constraints (e.g., being micromanaged by a superior). In other words, a job with high demands and low decision latitudes is considered a "high-strain" job in which employees tend to suffer poor physical and mental health. To combat the adverse effects of job demands, the demands-control model suggests increasing decision latitude through work design while employees face job demands so that job control can mitigate (or buffer) the adverse effects of job demands on their well-being (Ganster, 1989). According to van der Doef and Maes (1999), the strain hypothesis, in contrast to the buffering hypothesis, has received relatively consistent support. They found that only about half of reviewed studies support the buffering effect of job control on the negative relationship between job demands and well-being.

## 2.4.3   Demands–Control–Support Model

Subsequently, Johnson and Hall (1988) added a third job characteristic, coworker support, into the demands-control model, which became the demands-control-support model. Johnson and Hall found that lack of coworker support amplified the adverse impact on CVD prevalence for employees who experience high job demands and low decision latitudes. In other words, employees under work conditions with high job demands, low decision latitudes, and low coworker support (labeled as the *iso-strain hypothesis*) tend to have the highest CVD prevalence rate, compared with employees under other work conditions. Compared with the demands-control model, there have been relatively fewer studies that have investigated the demands-control-support model. Generally speaking, the iso-strain hypothesis has only been partially supported by 9 out of 18 studies reviewed by van der Doef and Maes (1999).

### Social Support

One source of social support – coworker support – has been incorporated into the demands-control-support model (Johnson & Hall, 1988). Yet, it is important to understand the roles of social support, by discussing types of social support and sources of social support further. With regard to types of social support, research in social support often differentiates between two types of social support: *emotional support behaviors* and *instrumental support behaviors*. Emotional support behaviors involve listening to others' work and non-work-related concerns, providing others with comfort and encouragement, talking about good things about the work, or making time for others, whereas instrumental support behaviors take the form of assisting with tasks; providing know-how, advice, and direction; or solving work problems. Mathieu et al. (2019) meta-analyzed relationship patterns of both support types, with work outcomes such as burnout, physical symptoms, job satisfaction, organizational commitment, turnover intention, or job performance. In general, they found that relationship patterns with the above outcomes were similar for both emotional and instrumental support, even though the behaviors of both types are different.

Furthermore, sources of support in the social support literature may include the organization, coworkers, supervisors, family and friends, etc. Compared with results for coworker support, meta-analytic results for supervisor support showed that it exhibits stronger positive effects on subordinates' well-being (Mathieu et al., 2019). This result highlights the important role of supervisor support, which is the focus of two preventive interventions described in Chapter 4 (see Sections 4.3.1 and 4.3.3).

Viswesvaran et al. (1999) meta-analyzed whether (1) social support reduces job strains, (2) job strains mobilize or elicit social support, (3) social support is mobilized in the presence of job stressors, (4) social support reduces perceived job stressors, and (5) social support buffers the adverse effects of perceived job stressors on employee well-being (or the relationship between perceived job stressors and employee well-being becomes weaker when social support increases). Overall, they found that social support was negatively related to job strains and job stressors, which supports the proposition that social support likely reduces job strains and mitigates perceived job stressors. These results were also supported in other meta-analyses (Luchman & González-Morales, 2013; Mathieu et al., 2019). Finally, Viswesvaran et al. (1999) and Mathieu et al. (2019) found evidence that social support buffers the relationship between perceived job stressors and job strains.

Although social support has often been found to mitigate adverse effects of job stressors on employee well-being, social support could exacerbate the negative effects (i.e., *reverse buffering effects*) as well. Under what circumstances could social support backfire unexpectedly? Beehr et al. (2010) indicated that social support may show reverse buffering effects when supportive interactions draw recipients' attention to stressful events or lead them to think bad things might happen at work again. Reverse buffering effects also happen when help from a supervisor makes a subordinate feel inadequate or incompetent, or when a close colleague tries to assist a recipient regardless of whether the recipient wants it or not.

Gray et al. (2020) further identified a list of unhelpful workplace social support practices in a qualitative study, and subsequently found in a survey that unhelpful workplace social support from a coworker is associated with increased negative emotions, dissatisfaction with coworkers, work-related burnout, and frustration. Furthermore, unhelpful workplace social support is related to lower competence-based self-esteem. Below is a summary of unhelpful workplace social support practices, based on Gray et al. (2020):

1. *Critical social support*: Supportive interactions make a recipient feel like they are being attacked, insulted, criticized, or put down. For instance, my colleague insults me when trying to help me improve my work.

2. *Imposed social support*: Social support is unwanted and forced on a recipient in a noncritical manner. For instance, my colleague tries to help by completing tasks for me that I want to do myself.

3. *Impractical social support*: Information offered by providers is impractical, unreasonable, or erroneous. For instance, my colleague provides vague solutions or bad advice regarding my work problems.

4. *Partial social support*: Social support is incomplete, imprecise, or unclear. For instance, my colleague gives me imprecise suggestions to solve my work problems.

5. *Undependable social support*: Support to complete a recipient's task is promised, but the provider fails to deliver in a reliable manner. For instance, my colleague does not follow through after offering to complete a task for me.

6. *Shortsighted social support*: Social support is offered by a colleague by taking over a task without teaching a recipient how to complete the task in the future. For instance, my colleague does my tasks for me rather than showing me how to do them.

7. *Uncomforting social support*: Supportive interactions make a recipient feel inadequate, incompetent, or worse about situations. For instance, my colleague is not helpful when trying to comfort me.

8. *Conflicting social support*: Support from different colleagues is conflicting or incompatible. For instance, my colleague offers advice that is not helpful, because it clashes with other advice I have received at work.

### 2.4.4   Job Demands–Resources (JD-R) Theory

In contrast to the effort–reward imbalance model (Siegrist, 1996), the demands–control model (Karasek, 1979), and the demandscontrol–support model (Johnson & Hall, 1988), the JD-R theory expands on the previous focus on a small set of job stressors (workload or conflicting demands) and job resources (e.g., job control, social support, or rewards). According to Bakker and Demerouti (2017), in the JD-R theory, *job demands* are broadly defined as physical, psychological, social, or organizational characteristics associated with any job in which employees are expected to constantly exert energy and efforts to regulate their actions to achieve goals at work. Resources consist of job resources and personal resources. *Job resources* are physical, psychological, social, or organizational characteristics associated with a job that assist employees to engage in work activities, achieve goals, and reduce job demands and their adverse impacts, as well as facilitate their personal growth, learning, and development. Examples of job resources include organizational support, supervisor support, coworker support, job control, appreciation, recognition, rewards, feedback, and opportunities for career development, as well as other motivational tasks, knowledge, and social and contextual characteristics (Morgeson & Humphrey, 2006). In contrast, *personal resources* are positive self-evaluations and beliefs about how much people can control their work, such as optimism, self-efficacy, self-esteem, work locus of control, assertiveness, resilience, or coping skills. References regarding self-reports of resource measures are listed in Appendix 2.

In addition, the JD-R theory simultaneously focuses on the process of health impairment (e.g., burnout) resulting from job demands, and the motivational process resulting from resources to increase work engagement and job performance (Bakker & Demerouti, 2014; Demerouti et al., 2001). Resources, particularly job resources, are expected to influence motivation to achieve goals and increase work engagement when job demands are high, which is similar to an increase of learning outcomes in a high demand–high control job as proposed by the demands–control model. Furthermore, the theory explicitly proposes joint effects of job demands and job resources.

The JD-R theory takes a top-down perspective to consider formal work design initiated by organizations, such as changing or improving a job or organizational characteristics, to enhance employee well-being. The unique aspect of the JD-R theory is that it also takes a bottom-up perspective – job crafting (Wrzesniewski & Dutton, 2001) – to conduct informal work designs initiated by employees with the goal of seeking job resources and challenges, as well as minimizing and optimizing demands. I will review job crafting and how it is implemented as a preventive intervention in Chapter 4 (Section 4.2).

# 3

# Job Stressors and Their Impacts

There has been an increase in occupational stress research over the past century, and accumulated findings have generated numerous meta-analyses since the 1980s. This chapter will describe the job stressors which have been widely studied in the occupational stress literature, and present available meta-analytical results pertaining to their main adverse effects on individual and organizational outcomes. Readers who are interested in potential moderators such as sample types; types of measures used; and types of industries, individual differences, etc., can refer to the corresponding references provided in each subsection below. To gauge the magnitude of effect pertaining to potential adverse effects, Cohen's recommendations (Cohen, 1988) are applied to interpret these estimated correlations: a small effect size ($r = 0.10$), a medium effect size ($r = 0.30$), and a large effect size ($r = 0.50$).

Job stressors covered in this chapter include role stressors (role conflict, role ambiguity, role overload, and illegitimate tasks), work–family conflict including work interference with family (WIF) and family interference with work (FIW), workload (including workplace telepressure), lack of control or autonomy, organizational constraints, organizational justice, organizational politics, and workplace mistreatment. References regarding self-reports of job stressors are provided in Appendix 3.

## 3.1    Role Conflict and Role Ambiguity

A *work role* consists of the pattern of work behaviors that people need to perform to achieve organizational goals and to meet management's expectations. For instance, the role of a mental health counselor likely consists of maintaining confidentiality of records about clients' treatments; assessing clients for suicidal thoughts, ideations, or attempts; motivating clients to express their feelings and thoughts; having discussions with clients about their lives; and helping clients develop awareness about themselves, etc. The circumstances disrupting a mental health counselor's role may be perceived as stressful if a counselor cannot achieve their goals.

*Role conflict* and *role ambiguity* are the job stressors that have been studied the most since role stress theory was introduced (see Section 2.1; Kahn et al., 1964). Role stressors tend to be chronic and create regulation uncertainty.

**Role conflict**    Role conflict arises when an individual receives incompatible or conflicting expectations, demands, or instructions about their role. Imagine a machine operator being asked to speed up production outputs by relaxing some safety regulations; in other words, being asked to do things differently. In another example, a software engineer might have to work under incompatible policies and guidelines (e.g., different approaches coming from a project manager and a team leader).

Role ambiguity happens when an individual's role is not clearly defined. **Role ambiguity** For instance, if an employee does not know what is expected of them, or works under vague directions or orders, then they cannot be certain about their responsibilities or authority.

The relationship between role stressors and individual and organizational outcomes has been reported in several meta-analytic studies. As described in Table 1, these meta-analytic results generally show that role stressors, particularly role ambiguity, tend to be associated with low commitment, engagement, and involvement toward jobs and organizations, as well as poor self-rated job performance. In addition, people who experience high levels of role ambiguity and conflict seem to receive relatively less feedback from others or less feedback about the tasks they perform. High role stressors are also related to high levels of job dissatisfaction, burnout, depression and anxiety, and physical symptoms, as well as strong intention to leave jobs. Role ambiguity, rather than role conflict, is positively related to absenteeism, although the effect size is small.

### 3.1.1   Role Overload

*Role overload* – a job stressor related to role stressors as well as to workload – reflects the extent to which people have inadequate organizational resources (e.g., time or personnel) or face constraints (e.g., lack of budget) and obstacles (e.g., excessive bureaucracy) while dealing with many responsibilities or work activities (Eatough et al., 2011). In high role overload circumstances, people may experience too many role demands without having adequate resources to meet those demands, find that their roles are too difficult to fulfill under constraints or obstacles, or feel as though their role demands overtax their capabilities. In a meta-analysis, Örtqvist and Wincent (2006) reported significant estimated correlations of role overload with emotional exhaustion (0.46), cynicism (0.18), and job dissatisfaction (0.07). The results of a meta-analysis by Eatough et al. (2011) further showed significant estimated correlations of role overload with role ambiguity (0.41), role conflict (0.62), and poor job performance (0.08).

### 3.1.2   Illegitimate Tasks

An *illegitimate task* – a recently identified role-related stressor – is any unreasonable or unnecessary task that violates the expected norms at work (Semmer et al., 2015). People may be faced with an *unreasonable task* when

**Table 1**
**Estimated Correlations of Role Ambiguity and Role Conflict With Individual and Organizational Outcomes**

| Outcome | Role ambiguity | Role conflict | Source |
|---|---|---|---|
| Absenteeism | .13 | −.02 | Jackson & Schuler (1985) |
| Cynicism | .31 | .40 | Alarcon (2011) |
| Depression | .29 | .32 | Schmidt et al. (2014) |
| Emotional exhaustion | .32 | .53 | Alarcon (2011) |
| Physical symptoms (cross-sectional analyses) | .15 | .27 | Nixon et al. (2011) |
| Physical symptoms (longitudinal analyses) | .17 | .10 | Nixon et al. (2011) |
| Reduced personal accomplishment | .31 | .18 | Alarcon (2011) |
| Tension/anxiety | .47 | .43 | Jackson & Schuler (1985) |
| Turnover intention | .29 | .34 | Jackson & Schuler (1985) |
| Commitment | −.41 | −.36 | Jackson & Schuler (1985) |
| Engagement | − | −.24 | Crawford et al. (2010) |
| Feedback from others | −.58 | −.31 | Jackson & Schuler (1985) |
| Feedback on tasks | −.41 | −.25 | Jackson & Schuler (1985) |
| Job involvement | −.44 | −.26 | Jackson & Schuler (1985) |
| Job satisfaction | −.34 | − | Abramis (1994) |
| | −.46 | −.48 | Jackson & Schuler (1985) |
| Job performance assessed by self | −.30 | − | Abramis (1994) |
| | −.30 | −.09 | Gilboa et al. (2008) |
| | −.37 | −.03 | Jackson & Schuler (1985) |
| | −.28 | −.06 | Tubre & Collins (2000) |
| Job performance assessed by others | −.10 | − | Abramis (1994) |
| | −.19 | −.12 | Gilboa et al. (2008) |
| | −.12 | −.11 | Jackson & Schuler (1985) |
| | −.20 | −.12 | Tubre & Collins (2000) |

asked to perform a task that should be done by someone else, should not be expected from them at all, or which goes too far. For instance, a supervisor might ask their staff to review contract language that is normally the supervisor's responsibility, or a manager might ask their assistant to buy movie tickets or make dinner reservations for them and their partner, pick up their laundry, walk their dog, and run other personal errands. Under normal circumstances, the above requested tasks are unreasonable because these tasks are outside of professional roles.

The second type of illegitimate task is an *unnecessary task*, which is observed when people question if it should have been done at all, could have been avoided, or could have been done with less effort. For instance, a worker might be asked to install unnecessary equipment, or a supervisor might ask their staff to use different pen colors for different types of projects. These tasks make no or little sense and tend to reflect poor management practices.

Overall, illegitimate tasks disrupt those in professional roles from achieving their goals. They become obstacles that prevent people from performing work activities well. These tasks may also be perceived as disrespectful and offensive, and can threaten professional identities and reduce people's sense of meaning and purpose (Semmer et al., 2015). A meta-analysis by Pindek et al. (2019) of a series of illegitimate tasks studies showed that illegitimate tasks are positively related to counterproductive work behaviors, feelings of resentment or irritation, anger, burnout, low self-esteem, high sleep fragmentation (i.e., frequently waking during sleep), depressive mood, job dissatisfaction, and negative emotions. Sonnentag and Lischetzke (2018) also reported their positive relationship with poor psychological detachment from work. Although both unreasonable and unnecessary tasks are associated with adverse outcomes, unreasonable tasks likely pose a greater risk to people's mental and physical well-being than unnecessary tasks (Pindek et al., 2019).

## 3.2    Work–Family Conflict

*Work-family conflict* is considered an interrole conflict in which people juggle incompatible or conflicting roles between work and family domains. Work and family domains are intertwined rather than independent from each other. The interrole conflict between family and work domains can happen from two directions: work-to-family conflict, and family-to-work conflict. *Work-to-family conflict* occurs when job demands (e.g., frequent business trips or long work hours) disrupt an individual's attention to family-related goals (e.g., attending a ball game or a child's graduation with family members). In other words, their work role interferes with with family role (WIF).

Similarly, *family-to-work conflict* occurs when family demands (e.g., taking care of aging parents or young children, or children's remote learning at home due to the COVID epidemic) disturb or interrupt an individual's activities in pursuing work-related goals. Thus their family role interferes with their work role (FIW).

There are two competing propositions about relationships of WIF and FIW with the correspondent adverse effects. The first proposition, the *cross-domain hypothesis*, suggests that WIF mainly affects the family domain, and FIW predominantly affects the work domain. The second proposition, the *matching hypothesis*, contends that the primary effects of work–family conflict occur in the domain in which causes of conflict originate. In other words, WIF is hypothesized to have stronger impacts on work-related outcomes than on family-related outcomes. Similarly, FIW is expected to have stronger effects on family-related outcomes than work-related outcomes. Evidence from a comprehensive meta-analysis (Amstad et al., 2011) generally supports the matching hypothesis.

Greenhaus and Beutell (1985) suggest that work–family conflict, whether WIF or FIW, often comes from three sources in one domain that interfere with the role in another domain. First, limited or inflexible time at work (e.g., shiftwork) or with family (e.g., large families) creates WIF or FIW. Second, experiencing job strains (e.g., being yelled at by a coworker) or family strains (e.g., having an argument with a spouse) causes WIF or FIW. Finally, behaviors exhibited at work (e.g., one is expected to be aggressive at work) and behaviors shown at home (e.g., one is expected to be warm with family members) are incompatible and lead to WIF or FIW. Both WIF and FIW inevitably disrupt actions, via regulation uncertainty, regulation obstacles, and overtaxing regulation.

It should be emphasized that work–family conflict is intertwined with stressors from both domains. Michel et al. (2011) meta-analyzed antecedents of work–family conflict and found that role conflict, role ambiguity, and role overload at work were stronger predictors of WIF than of FIW. Similarly, family role conflict, family role ambiguity, and family role overload were stronger predictors of FIW than of WIF. Support from sources (e.g., spouse or supervisor) in both domains also plays an important role in reducing inter-role conflict. Michel et al. (2011) also found that an increase in organizational support, supervisor support, and coworker support was associated with a decrease of WIF and FIW. In addition, an increase of family support and spousal support was associated with a decrease of WIF and FIW.

A meta-analysis by Goh et al. (2015) showed significant associations of work–family conflict with morbidity, mortality, perceived poor physical health, and perceived poor mental health. Work–family conflict was even more strongly related than secondhand smoke, to mortality and poorer physical and mental health.

A meta-analysis by Amstad et al. (2011) further showed that work–family conflict was often associated with three types of adverse consequences that are related to work (e.g., job satisfaction), family (e.g., family satisfaction), and unspecific domain (e.g., psychological strain). As described in Table 2, both WIF and FIW have been found to be associated with all three types of outcomes (i.e., job-related strain, family-related strain, or unspecific domain strain), although their relationships are generally stronger with outcomes of unspecific domain strain. These results further support the matching hypothesis in that both types of interrole conflict generally exhibit stronger relationships with outcomes of the same domain. In other words, WIF has stronger relationships with work-related outcomes than FIW. Similarly, FIW has stronger relationships with family-related outcomes than WIF.

**Table 2**
**Estimated Correlations of WIF and FIW With Three Types of Individual and Organizational Outcomes**

| Outcomes | WIF | FIW |
| --- | --- | --- |
| **Work-related outcome** | | |
| Career satisfaction | −.09 | – |
| Discretional behaviors that benefit other individuals and organizations | −.63 | −.54 |
| Job satisfaction | −.26 | −.13 |
| Job performance | −.11 | −.20 |
| Organizational commitment | −.17 | −.15 |
| Absenteeism | .03 | .09 |
| Burnout/exhaustion | .38 | .27 |
| Job-related strain | .49 | .28 |
| Turnover intention | .21 | .17 |
| **Family-related outcome** | | |
| Family satisfaction | −.18 | −.21 |
| Family function (performance) | −.18 | −.02 |
| Marital satisfaction | −.17 | −.29 |
| Family-related strain | .23 | .21 |
| **Domain-unspecific outcome** | | |
| Life satisfaction | −.31 | −.22 |
| Anxiety | .14 | .19 |
| Depression | .23 | .22 |
| Health problems | .28 | .24 |
| Psychological strain | .35 | .21 |
| Somatic/physical complaints | .29 | .14 |
| Stress | .54 | .39 |
| Substance use/abuse | .08 | .10 |

*Note.* FIW = family interference with work; WIF = work interference with family. Data from Amstad et al., 2011.

## 3.3    Workload

*Excessive workload*, either quantitative (i.e., high volume of work) or qualitative (i.e., difficult work), is one of the job stressors most frequently encountered, and the adverse impacts of workload on physical and mental health are well known in the occupational stress literature (Bowling et al., 2015). Workload can be an obstacle preventing workers from maintaining work and family relationships, and likely increases conflict between work and family. It also likely overtaxes people's ability to maintain mental well-being and physical health, because they are not able to detach themselves from work, or replenish energies drained at work. Workload also creates uncertainty about the ability to achieve goals when people need to complete daunting tasks within a limited time.

Japan's recently passed legislation, Work Style Reform Bill 2018, not only reflects Japan's extreme overwork culture, which has sometimes led to *karoshi* (overwork death), but also serves as a testimony to how workers have sometimes been treated unfairly and inhumanly by organizations. For instance, it was reported that the Subaru corporation did not pay the equivalent of US $7.08 million in overtime wages over a 2-year period to some 3,400 employees (Japan Times, 2019).

In the US, 45.5% of workers were working 41 hrs and longer per week across all industries, and 76.5% of workers in agriculture and related industries were working 41 hrs and longer each week as of January 2020 (US Bureau of Labor Statistics, 2021). It is not unusual, for instance, for construction or farm workers to leave home predawn to get to their job sites. Sometimes, they have no choice but to leave their families behind and live close to job sites that are far away from home for an indefinite period of time. During the summer, workers often spend long hours working, between sunrise and sunset. In addition, the prevalence of working long hours likely increases among people who hold multiple jobs. They account for 4.5% of 147 million employed people working more than one job in the US – for example, cleaning hotel rooms during the day and washing dishes in a restaurant at night.

Goh et al. (2015) reported significant associations of long work hours with morbidity, mortality, and perceived poor mental health. Working long hours is related more strongly than secondhand smoke, to mortality. Furthermore, three meta-analyses have reported the relationships between workload and individual and organizational outcomes (Bowling et al., 2015; Alarcon, 2011; Nixon et al., 2011). The estimated correlations they found are described in Table 3. Overall, workload was modestly related to physical health, as well as mental health outcomes, including depression, distress, fatigue, emotional exhaustion, and cynicism. Workload was also significantly related to absenteeism and turnover intention, as well as reduced personal accomplishment and affective commitment, although these effect sizes were small.

**Table 3**
**Estimated Correlations of Workload With Individual and Organizational Outcomes**

| Outcome | Workload | Source |
|---|---|---|
| Affective commitment | −.11 | Bowling et al. (2015) |
| Job satisfaction | −.22 | Bowling et al. (2015) |
| Absenteeism | .07 | Bowling et al. (2015) |
| Depression | .22 | Bowling et al. (2015) |
| Distress | .26 | Bowling et al. (2015) |
| Fatigue | .30 | Bowling et al. (2015) |
| Emotional exhaustion | .49 | Alarcon (2011) |
|  | .47 | Bowling et al. (2015) |
| Cynicism | .31 | Alarcon (2011) |
|  | .33 | Bowling et al. (2015) |
| Reduced personal accomplishment | .11 | Alarcon (2011) |
|  | .12 | Bowling et al. (2015) |
| Physical symptoms | .30 | Bowling et al. (2015) |
| Physical symptoms (cross-sectional analyses) | .22 | Nixon et al. (2011) |
| Physical symptoms (longitudinal analyses) | .16 | Nixon et al. (2011) |
| Poor global health | .27 | Bowling et al. (2015) |
| Poor mental well-being | .30 | Bowling et al. (2015) |
| Strain | .36 | Bowling et al. (2015) |
| Turnover intention | .16 | Bowling et al. (2015) |

### 3.3.1  Workplace Telepressure

A new form of workload – *workplace telepressure* – results from advancement of information and communication technologies. It arises when using asynchronous communications, such as voice mails, emails, and texts, which are supposed to offer flexibility and convenience, but instead often require immediate attention and responses. This type of pressure can also result from synchronous communications, such as via Zoom or Microsoft Teams, occurring in different time zones. People are often expected to quickly make decisions and respond to inquiries and requests from clients, coworkers, or superiors. They may feel the need to engage in work and obligated to commit to an organization by being continuously connected to work. It is not surprising that people experiencing telepressure tend to report high workload, physical fatigue, and cognitive weariness. They tend to have difficultly detaching from work, experience poor sleep quality, and report high absenteeism (Barber & Santuzzi, 2015).

## 3.4    Lack of Control or Autonomy

A core job characteristic, *job autonomy* shapes employees' experiences regarding the meaningfulness of their work via providing them with degrees of freedom, discretion, or control to do their work (Hackman & Oldham, 1976). It is one of the key components of the demands–control model (Karasek, 1979) and one of the important job resources proposed by the JD-R theory (Bakker & Demerouti, 2017). According to O*NET (2021), certain job characteristics allow employees to make decisions that affect other people, financial resources, and/or the image and reputation of organizations, or they are structured in a manner that allows employees to make decisions without supervision (Li et al., 2019).

In addition to being one of the major job characteristics and resources, organizational policies, rules, and management styles affect how people are empowered to structure or control their work environment or work activities. As a result, even people who hold a job with a high degree of autonomy may be managed differently across organizations, and they may have different perceived control across organizations. For instance, some people may experience little or no freedom or flexibility to help their clients, solve problems, or save money for their organizations, because of organizational policies, rules, or management's preferences, even if they have figured out obvious solutions.

Goh et al. (2015) revealed significant associations of low levels of job control with morbidity, mortality, perceived poor physical health, and perceived poor mental health. They also found that low job control is more likely than secondhand smoke to affect mortality. In addition, the relationships between job control and individual and organizational outcomes have been reported in several meta-analyses. As shown in Table 4, most of the estimated correlations were moderate in magnitude. Overall, people perceiving relatively high levels of job control tended to perform jobs well, and were more satisfied, committed, and involved with their jobs. In contrast, people experiencing relatively low levels of job control tended to be absent from work, to leave their jobs, and reported more physical symptoms and emotional distress. Spector (1986) also reported strong associations between lack of control and role conflict (0.41) and role ambiguity (0.42). Although the benefit of empowering employees is evident from these meta-analyses, people who take charge of tasks (e.g., improve procedures or institute new work methods) likely experience resource drain (e.g., time, attention, energy) and may have difficulty unwinding after work when tasks are less enjoyable or important (Cangiano et al., 2021).

**Table 4**
**Estimated Correlations of Lack of Control or Autonomy With Individual and Organizational Outcomes**

| Outcome | Lack of control | Source |
|---|---|---|
| Commitment | −.32 | Spector (1986) |
| Job involvement | −.54 | Spector (1986) |
| Job performance | −.25 | Spector (1986) |
| Job satisfaction | −.44 | Spector (1986) |
| Absenteeism | .22 | Spector (1986) |
| Emotional distress | .32 | Spector (1986) |
| Cynicism | .29 | Park et al. (2014) |
| Emotional exhaustion | .20 | Park et al. (2014) |
| Reduced personal accomplishment | .36 | Park et al. (2014) |
| Physical symptoms | .34 | Spector (1986) |
| Physical symptoms (cross-sectional analyses) | .07 | Nixon et al. (2011) |
| Physical symptoms (longitudinal analyses) | .14 | Nixon et al. (2011) |
| Psychological strain | .23 | Gonzalez-Mulé et al. (2021) |
| Turnover intention | .23 | Spector (1986) |
| Turnover | .25 | Spector (1986) |

## 3.5    Organizational Constraints

*Organizational constraints* are work conditions that interfere with people's ability to perform their tasks at work (Peters & O'Connor, 1980). These constraints may include, but are not limited to, a lack of job-related information, material and supplies, budgetary support, task preparation and training, time availability, or physical aspects of the work environment. Organizational constraints, which were one of the most-often-mentioned job stressors by American and Chinese employees in a study by Liu et al. (2007), likely create *uncertainty* (e.g., uncertainty about whether there is budgetary support or needed personnel available to achieve goals), *obstacles* (e.g., if equipment, physical spaces, or job-related information is unavailable or is not adequately provided), or be *overtaxing* (e.g., inadequate training is given to perform work activities). Imagine nurses caring for COVID-19 patients without adequate personal protective equipment or sufficient time to recover from each shift. It is likely that they will experience frustration, anxiety, anger, fear, dissatisfaction, or exhaustion, because their work activities are disrupted or disturbed.

**Table 5**
**Estimated Correlations of Organizational Constraints With Individual and Organizational Outcomes**

| Outcome | Self-report | Other-report[a] | Source |
|---|---|---|---|
| Commitment | −.32 | – | Pindek & Spector (2016) |
| Job satisfaction | −.39 | −.24 | Pindek & Spector (2016) |
| | −.32 | – | Villanova & Roman (1993) |
| Job performance assessed by others | −.24 | – | Gilboa et al. (2008) |
| Job performance | −.14 | – | Villanova & Roman (1993) |
| Well-being/mental health | −.33 | – | Pindek & Spector (2016) |
| Absenteeism | .27 | – | Pindek & Spector (2016) |
| Anxiety | .50 | – | Pindek & Spector (2016) |
| Counterproductive work behavior | .43 | .29 | Pindek & Spector (2016) |
| Emotional exhaustion | .42 | – | Pindek & Spector (2016) |
| Frustration | .51 | – | Pindek & Spector (2016) |
| Interpersonal aggression | .45 | – | Pindek & Spector (2016) |
| | .30 | – | Hershcovis et al. (2007) |
| Lateness | .38 | – | Pindek & Spector (2016) |
| Negative emotions | .47 | .24 | Pindek & Spector (2016) |
| Organizational targeted aggression | .36 | – | Hershcovis et al. (2007) |
| Physical symptoms | .40 | – | Pindek & Spector (2016) |
| | .33 | – | Nixon et al. (2011) |
| Sabotage | .38 | – | Pindek & Spector (2016) |
| Stress | .41 | .39 | Pindek & Spector (2016) |
| Theft | .34 | – | Pindek & Spector (2016) |
| Turnover intention | .39 | .23 | Pindek & Spector (2016) |

*Note.* [a]Organizational constraints were reported by either a coworker or a supervisor.

There have been several meta-analyses reporting correlations between organizational constraints and individual and organizational outcomes. As shown in Table 5, organizational constraints have been found to be strongly related to an array of individual and organizational outcome variables. For instance, people experiencing high levels of constraints often report high levels of physical symptoms, negative emotions, job dissatisfaction, frustration, anxiety, stress, and emotional exhaustion. Foremost among these, the relationship between organizational constraints and counterproductive behaviors, sabotage, interpersonal aggression, organizational targeted aggression, or theft are alarming, considering the direct and indirect costs associated with these types of behavior.

## 3.6   Organizational Justice

*Organizational justice,* or fair treatment at work, reflects whether or not people are treated with respect, dignity, and politeness. These experiences emerge from three forms of organizational justice that are appraised by people: perceived fairness of outcomes (e.g., rewards) being distributed and allocated (*distributive justice*), perceived fairness of the processes that have been developed and implemented to reach decisions about distribution or allocation of outcomes (*procedural justice*), and fairness of interpersonal treatment and communication by management (*interactional justice*).

Perceived injustice or unfairness regarding how outcome allocations are determined or executed is a major job stressor, because it often disrupts regulation of actions while pursuing goals. These perceptions create uncertainty because people are not sure if they will receive outcomes (e.g., rewards) based on their work activities or efforts. In addition, these perceptions become obstacles to motivation, and prevent people from making efforts to complete work assignments.

Procedures are considered fair when the process of allocating outcomes is consistent across people and over time, decision makers' self-interests or biases are suppressed and prevented, the allocation process is compatible with moral values and ethical standards, allocation procedures are accurate, allocation decisions are correctable should unfair decisions occur, and the needs and values of all involved parties are represented (Cohen-Charash & Spector, 2001).

Procedural justice is often viewed as more important than distributive justice because the former has broader implications and impacts. In contrast, the latter mainly focuses on the perceived fairness of a particular outcome. This view has generally been supported by two meta-analyses (Cohen-Charash & Spector, 2001; Colquitt et al., 2001), which showed stronger correlations overall of outcomes with procedural justice than with distributive justice. Finally, past research has consistently shown that the adverse effects of distributive justice become weaker when people view the process and procedure as fair (Cropanzano & Wright, 2011).

There has been a debate around whether interactional justice is part of procedural justice (Colquitt et al., 2001). However, evidence suggests that procedural justice can be distinguished from interactional justice, with the former emphasizing exchanges between workers and their senior management or organizations, and the latter emphasizing exchanges between workers and their supervisors (Cropanzano et al., 2002). Interactional justice has been divided into two types of interpersonal treatment: *interpersonal justice* and *informational justice*. According to Colquitt et al., interpersonal justice refers to how people are treated with respect by authorities who execute allocation procedures, and informational justice reflects how explanations are adequately conveyed to people regarding why allocation procedures are implemented in certain ways.

Greenberg (2010) reviewed the literature from sociology, medicine, and psychology, and concluded that people who perceive unfair treatment at work are likely to suffer mental and physical illness. According to Siegrist's effort–reward imbalance model (Section 2.4.1; see Siegrist, 1996), people experience negative emotions and psychological distress when they work hard yet receive few rewards in return. Siegrist also provided epidemiological evidence regarding the positive relationship between perceived inequity and cardiovascular illness. Furthermore, Greenberg suggested that perceived injustice as well as negative emotions are likely to trigger unhealthy behaviors such as a sedentary lifestyle, smoking, or alcohol consumption. Goh et al. (2015) further supported Greenberg's contention, and reported significant associations of organizational injustice with morbidity, mortality, perceived poor physical health, and perceived poor mental health. Furthermore, exposure to high levels of organizational injustice is more strongly related than secondhand smoke, to morbidity and poor mental health.

Cohen-Charash and Spector (2001) postulated that perceived injustice likely leads to negative emotions toward, and negative perceptions of, the organization, and people are likely to engage in counterproductive behaviors or retaliation, quit their jobs, and disengage with discretionary behaviors that benefit others in organizations. Furthermore, unfair treatment leads people to exert less effort at work, so that they can restore feelings of equity.

Two meta-analyses have provided clear evidence of the adverse effects of organizational injustice. Cohen-Charash and Spector (2001) reported estimated intercorrelations among distributive justice, procedural justice, and interactional justice, ranging from 0.46 to 0.55. Colquitt et al. (2001) reported estimated intercorrelations among distributive justice, procedural justice, interpersonal justice, and informational justice, ranging from 0.38 to 0.66. As shown in Table 6 and Table 7, the magnitudes of the estimated correlations with organizational justice dimensions were either moderate or strong for most outcome variables. Overall, people who perceive fairness tend to be more satisfied and committed, have better relationships with supervisors, and trust their organizations and supervisors more strongly. In contrast, people who perceive unfair treatment tend to experience higher levels of negative emotions, have stronger intentions to leave their jobs, and display withdrawal behaviors more frequently (e.g., absenteeism and turnover).

Finally, perceived organizational injustice is generally related to more counterproductive work behaviors or negative reactions, poorer job performance, and fewer discretional behaviors that benefit organizations and other individuals. However, these correlations were small or modest in magnitude.

**Table 6**
**Estimated Correlations of Organizational Justice Dimensions With Individual and Organizational Outcomes**

| Outcome | Distributive justice | Procedural justice | Interactional justice |
|---|---|---|---|
| Counterproductive work behaviors | −.22 | −.28 | − |
| Conflict with others | −.18 | −.19 | − |
| Negative emotions | −.27 | −.32 | − |
| Turnover intention | −.40 | −.40 | −.24 |
| Affective commitment | .47 | .50 | .38 |
| Continuance commitment | − | −.22 | −.12 |
| Discretional behaviors that benefit other individuals and organizations | .25 | .23 | − |
| Discretional behaviors that benefit other individuals | − | .03 | − |
| Discretional behaviors that benefit organizations | − | .22 | − |
| Job satisfaction | .47 | .43 | .41 |
| Leader–member exchange quality | .27 | .37 | .67 |
| Normative commitment | − | .41 | − |
| Pay satisfaction | .62 | .48 | − |
| Recommend the organization to others | − | .53 | − |
| Satisfaction with supervisor | .58 | .57 | .52 |
| Satisfaction with management | .27 | .27 | − |
| Satisfaction with union | .45 | .52 | − |
| Satisfaction with performance evaluation | .63 | − | − |
| Trust in organization | .43 | .48 | .35 |
| Trust in supervisor | .55 | .65 | − |
| Trust – other justice source | .33 | .49 | − |

*Note.* Data from Cohen-Charash & Spector, 2001.

**Table 7**
**Estimated Correlations of Organizational Justice Dimensions With Individual and Organizational Outcomes**

| Outcome | Distributive justice | Procedural justice | Interpersonal justice | Informational justice |
|---|---|---|---|---|
| Discretional behaviors that benefit other individuals | .15 | .22 | .29 | .26 |
| Discretional behaviors that benefit organizations | .25 | .27 | – | – |
| Evaluation of supervisor | .59 | .64 | .62 | .65 |
| Evaluation of management in general | .37 | .42 | .23 | .47 |
| Job performance | .15 | .36 | .03 | .13 |
| Job satisfaction | .56 | .62 | .35 | .43 |
| Negative reactions (theft, retaliatory behaviors) | −.30 | −.31 | −.35 | −.33 |
| Organizational commitment | .51 | .57 | .19 | .29 |
| Satisfaction with pay, promotion, or performance evaluation | .61 | .48 | – | .30 |
| Trust | .57 | .61 | – | .51 |
| Withdrawal behaviors (absenteeism, turnover) | −.50 | -.46 | −.02 | −.24 |

*Note.* Data from Colquitt et al., 2001.

## 3.7    Organizational Politics

Organizations are political entities in which certain policies or procedures are influenced or controlled, power and resources are competed for, and decisions about priority goals are made through varying degrees of political behaviors that involve negotiation, bargaining, or competitive tactics. Thus, political behaviors are likely seen at work when people exercise influence tactics to obtain expected outcomes that are not sanctioned by organizations, or to use nonsanctioned influence tactics to obtain sanctioned outcomes (Mayes & Allen, 1977). For instance, a foreman might abuse their authority by threatening their crew for not following safety regulations to meet production goals, whereas another supervisor might motivate their crew to follow safety regulations to meet production goals. Under normal circumstances, the former types of behavior are sanctioned by organizations and considered dysfunctional political behaviors, in contrast to the latter types of behaviors, which are likely functional to organizations.

Another example is when rewards or promotions are politically applied by a manager to their team members, or when a performance review an individual receives mainly reflects their supervisor's favoritism, rather than actual performance standards. These types of political behaviors are considered dysfunctional to organizations as well.

Dysfunctional political behaviors are a widely observed job stressor across different levels of organizations, and organizational politics inevitably create uncertainty or become obstacles that disrupt how people regulate their actions to achieve goals. When people are exposed to frequent dysfunctional political behaviors at work, according to PE fit theory (Section 2.3), they may feel misfit with the political environment if they do not get involved in the political processes, and develop unfavorable and uncertain feelings toward their job outlooks and organizations. Some may avoid political work environments by being less involved in their work, committing less to their organizations, or seeking out other jobs that better fit their preferences. Those individuals who get involved in organizational politics, which can be a risky, uncertain, and ambiguous process, likely experience high levels of anxiety and arousal, as well as other negative emotions (Ferris & Kacmar, 1992).

A meta-analysis by Chang et al. (2009) showed that organizational politics was strongly correlated to role ambiguity (0.52) and role conflict (0.58). In addition, it was strongly associated with decreased commitment and job satisfaction, and increased psychological strain and turnover intention. However, the strength of its relationship with job performance and discretional behaviors to benefit others or organizations was modest. Estimated correlations are shown in Table 8.

**Table 8**
**Estimated Correlations of Organizational Politics With Individual and Organizational Outcomes**

| Outcome | Organizational politics |
| --- | --- |
| Affective commitment | −.54 |
| Job satisfaction | −.57 |
| Job performance | −.20 |
| Discretional behaviors that benefit other individuals | −.16 |
| Discretional behaviors that benefit organizations | −.20 |
| Psychological strain | .48 |
| Turnover intention | .43 |

Note. Data from Chang et al., 2009.

## 3.8    Workplace Mistreatment

Being *mistreated at work* by others, including coworkers, customers, subordinates, or supervisors, is considered a major job stressor that disrupts an individual's capacity to regulate their actions. People experiencing mistreatment are uncertain if their work activities matter to their jobs. Mistreatments themselves are clearly obstacles that prevent people from engaging in their daily work activities and maximizing their talents to excel, and often lead to anxiety, frustration, resentment, depression, low self-esteem, burnout, negative reactions, withdrawal behaviors, or even hopelessness. Being exposed to mistreatments further drain individuals' energies and resources and overtaxes their capacities to deal with mistreatment incidents and sources of mistreatment incidents while engaging in work activities at the same time.

Workplace mistreatment reflects the dark side of human behaviors in organizations. Prevalence of workplace mistreatment is often shaped by an organizational climate – *mistreatment climate* – which refers to organizational policies, procedures, and practices that either encourage, ignore, or deter mistreatment behaviors (Yang et al., 2014). A meta-analysis by Yang et al. (2014) has shown that a climate that deters workplace mistreatment is strongly associated with increased job satisfaction and organizational commitment, and a decrease in turnover intention, emotional strains, physical strains, and physical and nonphysical aggression, as well as incidents of incivility.

There are different types of workplace mistreatment, such as social undermining, incivility, workplace ostracism, bullying, mobbing, workplace aggression, interpersonal conflict, deviance, antisocial behavior, emotional abuse, abusive supervision, harassment, and discrimination. Hershcovis (2011) suggested that the above mistreatment behaviors can generally be classified via one or more dimensions: intensity (minor to severe), frequency, types of perpetrators (e.g., abusive supervisor or bullying coworkers), intention attribution (e.g., nonintentional acts, ambiguous intent, or intentional acts), as well as outcomes to be affected (e.g., relationship, reputation, or success).

For instance, *social undermining* occurs when individuals' abilities to pursue success are intentionally hindered by others; *workplace ostracism* occurs when individuals are inappropriately ignored, rejected, or excluded by others; *uncivil behaviors* are low-intensity verbal or nonverbal deviant behaviors with an ambiguous intent to hurt people; and *bullying* involves negative acts directed at targeted individuals repeatedly and regularly over time. Regardless of the type of workplace mistreatment, being mistreated at work is a risk to individuals' psychological and physical well-being, and tends to lead to job dissatisfaction, poor job performance, frequent absence, high turnover intention, low commitment to the organization (Hershcovis, 2011; Nielsen & Einarsen, 2012), and even retaliatory behaviors to reduce the harmful effects of mistreatment (Liang et al., 2022).

Hassard et al. (2018b) estimated that annual costs attributed to workplace aggression range from US $114.64 million to $35.9 billion (adjusted to 2014

US dollar rates) across five countries (Australia, Italy, Spain, the UK, and the US). Similarly, Hassard et al. (2019) estimated that the costs attributed to severe workplace violence (e.g., homicide and assault), primarily in the US, vary from US $2.36 million to $55.86 billion (adjusted to 2017 US dollar rates). A 2021 RAND report (Morral et al., 2021) estimated that sexual assault and sexual harassment in the US military are associated with 2,000 victims and 8,000 victims, respectively, most of whom left the military over a 28-month period following the incidents, yielding a premature and preventable loss of a minimum of 16,000 labor-years. These data clearly point out the burdens and costs for active-duty victims (e.g., psychological health, physical health, treatment, career, and financial hardships such as loss of post-retirement compensation) and the US military (turnover, recruitment, reputation, image, training, and military readiness).

A comprehensive meta-analysis that covered different types of mistreatment behaviors from the victim's perspective highlighted three major observations from past research (Bowling & Beehr, 2006). First, people being mistreated may attribute causes of mistreatment to perpetrators or organizations, and they may reciprocate with hostile reactions (e.g., counterproductive work behavior). Second, job stressors experienced by people who are mistreated may be experienced by perpetrators too. It may explain in part why perpetrators exposed to high levels of job stressors such as organizational constraints, distributive and procedural injustice, and interpersonal conflict (Hershcovis et al., 2007) likely experience frustrations and other negative emotions, and lash out with negative reactions toward other people. Third, people being mistreated suffer from a wide variety of ill health and poor well-being. A summary of Bowling and Beehr's (2006) meta-analysis results is displayed in Table 9.

Paul Spector (2021), an eminent occupational health psychologist, has succinctly summarized the steps involved in building a healthier work organization. They include having proper staffing and sound management that builds a psychologically safe workplace in which employees are empowered to perform tasks, are treated fairly and respectfully, and are supported in balancing their work versus family and nonwork life. In a healthy organization, psychological hazards (e.g., role stressors, workload, organizational constraints, organizational politics, and mistreatment) are monitored, controlled, reduced, and eliminated by applying human resources analytics and preventive management initiatives. Promising practices have been recommended by Total Worker Health (US National Institute for Occupational Safety and Health, 2022).

Each job stressor described in this chapter does not necessarily occur independent of other job stressors. Past research has consistently shown that job stressors are often correlated with one another. It is not surprising, for instance, that work–family conflict is related to various job demands (Ilies et al., 2015). In the next and final chapter, I will describe evidence-based prevention strategies that can be applied to address various job stressors in order to build a psychologically safe and healthy workplace.

**Table 9**
**Estimated Correlations of Workplace Mistreatment With Job Stressors, Individual and Organizational Outcomes**

| Job stressors and outcomes | Workplace mistreatment |
|---|---|
| **Stressor** | |
| Role conflict | .44 |
| Role ambiguity | .30 |
| Role overload | .28 |
| Organizational constraints | .53 |
| Lack of control | .25 |
| Organizational injustice | .35 |
| **Outcome** | |
| Anxiety | .31 |
| Burnout | .39 |
| Depression | .34 |
| Frustration | .40 |
| Negative emotions | .46 |
| Poor self-esteem | .21 |
| Life dissatisfaction | .21 |
| Job dissatisfaction | .39 |
| Psychological strains | .35 |
| Physical symptoms | .31 |
| Counterproductive work behavior | .37 |
| Turnover intention | .35 |
| Absenteeism | .06 |
| Organizational commitment | −.36 |
| Job performance | −.08 |
| Discretional behaviors that benefit other individuals or organizations | −.03 |

*Note.* Data from Bowling & Beehr, 2006.

# 4

# Preventive Interventions

Occupational stress management interventions are commonly classified as primary, secondary, or tertiary interventions. *Primary intervention programs* are proactive and preventive, aiming to alter job stressors and counter job strains. Relatively few empirical studies in occupational stress management fall into this category.

*Secondary intervention programs* aim at reducing employees' severe symptoms (e.g., depression) or modifying their reactions to perceived job stressors. The goals of these programs are to assist employees to regulate their emotions, reduce their experienced strains, and improve their behaviors. These programs are the most reported occupational stress management programs in the occupational stress literature (Bellarosa & Chen, 1997). Examples of these programs include relaxation, deep breathing, mindfulness training, physical fitness, cognitive behavior therapy, cognitive-behavioral skill training, meditation, assertiveness training, stress inoculation, journaling, reflection, effective coping skills, emotional regulation (e.g., anger control), and time management. Readers who are interested in meta-analytic evaluations of resilience intervention programs (mixed with cognitive behavior therapy), wellness programs, and mindfulness intervention can refer to a number of studies (Bartlett et al., 2019; Cores et al., 2021; Joyce et al., 2018; Parks & Steelman, 2008; Richardson & Rothstein, 2008; Vanhove et al., 2016).

*Goal: Symptom reduction and behavior change*

*Tertiary intervention programs* are designed to treat employees' health conditions (e.g., mental disorders or posttraumatic stress disorder). For example, return-to-work programs, employee assistance programs, occupational therapy, or medical treatment can address various health conditions.

*Goal: Treatment of health conditions*

In the remaining sections, five types of organizational stress management intervention programs will be described, which focus on recovery from work, self-initiated work redesign (i.e., job crafting), work–family balance, mistreatment prevention, and organization-initiated work design. These programs are considered primary intervention programs. They are preventive and proactive in nature, although some of them include techniques such as mindfulness, resilience building, relaxation, exercises, and emotional regulation, which are typically applied in secondary intervention programs. From a practical viewpoint, organizational stress management with a focus on proactive prevention would likely have greater impacts on employees' physical and psychological well-being.

Organizational stress management intervention programs can be modified and applied to individuals, supervisors, or organizations to address a wide variety of job stressors. These programs have been developed based on theoretical frameworks with robust and rigorous research designs (i.e., multiple follow-up assessments and quasi or true field experiments). Furthermore, they have been successfully replicated. Finally, these programs specifically and directly address workplace issues experienced by employees.

Most of these programs apply psychological principles, such as *goal-setting theory* or *social learning the*ory, to increase participants' motivation to achieve goals, and to raise self-efficacy to achieve goals (Locke & Latham, 2002). According to Locke and Latham (2002), goals change and improve human behaviors through providing clear direction, energizing efforts to pursue goals, encouraging a person to be persistent, and motivating them to take action. To effectively apply goal-setting theory to motivate training participants to change or improve their behaviors, trainers often encourage trainees to set goals that are specific (observable or measurable), to commit to goals by setting specific target dates to achieve them, and to make goals realistic and challenging.

Training participants who observe successful or effective behaviors of other participants in a group discussion, or who are persuaded by other participants, are likely to increase their self-efficacy and motivation to engage in trained behaviors (Bandura, 1991). In addition, most of the programs apply strategies recommended by organizational training literature (Noe & Colquitt, 2002) to facilitate learning and training transfer. These strategies include role play, timely feedback, or distributed practice between training sessions.

## 4.1    Promoting Recovery From Work

Employees experience strains attributed to job stressors they encounter each day. In addition, employees constantly regulate the expression of their emotions (types, intensity, frequency, and duration) under different circumstances, while interacting with supervisors, colleagues, customers, or other individuals they encounter at work. This experience can be quite exhausting and energy draining! Often, they have to suppress their felt emotions at work to meet rules required or expected by organizations. The dissonance between felt emotions and required emotions is inevitably prolonged after work. That dissonance has been found in a meta-analysis to be positively associated with burnout, psychological strain, and psychosomatic complaints as well as poor job attitude (Hülsheger & Schewe, 2011).

Furthermore, there is an increasing trend around the globe for employees to work during leisure time, check and process work emails or voice mails during off-job time, and delay or give up vacation leave. Facing these challenges, employees struggle to recover during off-job time or breaks at work, because they cannot mentally switch off these experiences, unwind the tension, or stop repetitive negative emotions (e.g., rumination). Failure to recover from work means that employees are less likely to replenish depleted resources, gain new resources, or stop resources loss before they go back to work.

There are four different but essential recovery experiences that employees can practice during off-job time or breaks at work through a variety of activities (Sonnentag & Fritz, 2007) to increase psychological detachment, relaxation, mastery, and control. *Psychological detachment* refers to a person's ability to physically or mentally distance and disengage themselves from their jobs. People with a high level of psychological detachment tend not to be occupied by work duties, do not think about work-related problems or challenges, and do not engage in job related activities. *Relaxation* is a mental state characterized by ease, calm, and low sympathetic activation. This state tends to reduce physical and mental arousal or activation of the psychophysiological system, increase positive affect, and reduce job strain experiences.

*Mastery* generally occurs when people engage in non-job-related activities that provide intellectual challenges or learning opportunities. Although activities that foster mastery may put additional demands on people, these activities do not necessarily overtax their capabilities or become burdens. Instead, these activities help people acquire news skills, increase their sense of competency, and distract them from any negative experience attributed to work. Finally, *control* refers to a sense of autonomy – people can decide for themselves when and how to spend their time, and engage in off-work activities that meet their needs.

Two meta-analyses highlight the important role of recovery experiences in relation to increased mental well-being, positive affect, life satisfaction, vigor, and decreased negative affect and fatigue (Bennett et al., 2018; Steed et al., 2021). For readers' convenience, key strategies applicable to fostering psychological detachment, relaxation, mastery, and control experiences are summarized in Box 1.

> **Recovery experiences replenish depleted resources, gain new resources, or stop resources loss**

> **Box 1**
> **Strategies to Foster Four Different Recovery Experiences**
>
> **Detachment Experiences**
>
> - Triage and prioritize urgent and important work and home demands.
> - Use skills and availability of other people to help maintain work and home boundary.
> - Use technology to facilitate boundary between work and home domain.
> - Leave office materials at work.
> - Get away from home (e.g., retreat to a remote area).
> - Block off segments of time.
> - Erect physical borders or physical distance between work and nonwork domains.
> - Separate work artifacts from home artifacts (e.g., home calendars, keys, photos, mail).
> - Set up expectations in advance of off-job hours (e.g., no email or voice mail contact).
> - Engage in physical activities (dancing, jogging, swimming, etc.).
> - Socialize with friends.
> - Use Ellis's ABC thought awareness exercise to regulate emotions (Ellis, 1977).

- Reduce emotional responses toward a stressful event by changing the appraisal of the event (e.g., reappraise the situation or consider resources available to deal with the event).
- Reduce emotional responses toward a stressful event by using attentional deployment (i.e., shift attention to positive and enjoyable events).
- Reduce stressors via problem solving.
- Reduce job demands through work design.
- Practice sleep hygiene to improve sleep.
- Increase resources through work design.
- Engage in positive work reflection (e.g., write down three good job-related events that happened at work that day and explain why these positive events occurred).
- Reduce rumination via taking different perspectives.
- Reduce rumination via practicing mindfulness (e.g., a combination of meditation, total body awareness, yoga, etc.).
- Reduce rumination via practicing distraction (e.g., purposely focus on positive events or activities such as watching a movie).
- Reduce rumination via reappraising situations or sources of job strains (e.g., view it as a personal challenge or opportunity to grow).

**Relaxation Experiences**

- Exercise, yoga, walking, and practicing muscle relaxation, meditation, or mindfulness.
- Take a light walk during leisure time or lunch breaks at work.
- Listen to music.
- Practice sleep hygiene.
- Take work breaks.
- Reduce social demands such as attending formal parties.

**Mastery Experiences**

- Learn a new language.
- Learn a new hobby.
- Volunteer for non-job-related tasks (e.g., sort and pack boxes of food for distribution in a foodbank or deliver meals).
- Learn a new sport.
- Do creative work.
- Climb a mountain or hike a trail.

**Control Experiences**

- Decide on an off-work schedule.
- Manage time.
- Spend leisure time on activities that best fit your preferences.
- Cut down leisure activities that are incongruent with personal goals.
- Cut down leisure activities that are stressful.
- Leave time for more preferred activities.
- Identify different options to increase control during off-work time.

Adapted from Bartlett et al., 2019; Grandey & Melloy, 2017; Hahn et al., 2011; Hülsheger et al., 2015; Karabinski et al., 2021; Kreiner et al., 2009; Sonnentag & Fritz, 2007; and Verbeek et al., 2019.

Two meta-analyses have investigated a wide variety of recovery intervention programs (Karabinski et al., 2021; Verbeek et al., 2019) that emphasize one or more of the four recovery experiences. Because detachment is a prototypical recovery experience and has shown relatively stronger relationships with outcomes (Sonnentag & Fritz, 2015), detachment has often been a focus in interventions. Thirty detachment intervention studies reported in a meta-analysis by Karabinski et al. (2021) showed an overall moderate effect size in increasing detachment and positive work-related thinking, decreasing negative work-related thinking, and improving emotion regulation. There are diverse interventions that apply different strategies to foster recovery experiences; below a recovery intervention that covers four recovery experiences is described and how that intervention is implemented.

Hahn et al. (2011) conducted a recovery intervention program with four modules containing educational materials and exercises. The program was conducted in two different sessions, 1 week apart. The intervention applied principles of goal-setting theory and social learning theory to motivate and increase training participants' self-efficacy.

In the first training session, two modules were delivered. The first module aimed to increase control experiences by training participants how to control their activities during their off-job time. In a small group, participants shared their own off-work activities that increased control experiences and discussed obstacles that prevented them from spending more time on activities they liked and less time on activities they did not like. Then, participants learned and practiced setting specific and concrete goals regarding improving control experiences. In addition, they learned time management techniques so that they could better manage or control their off-job time.

The second module aimed to improve psychological detachment from work. Participants learned about the concept of psychological detachment, and strategies to distance themselves from work. They also shared their own leisure activities during which they forgot about their work. At the end of the first training session, participants were instructed to write down the key learning points they had taken from both modules. They also wrote down their goals to improve their recovery experiences until the second training session. Their goals were documented on a poster too.

At the beginning of the second training session, participants discussed whether they had met the goals they set up in the previous week. They shared circumstances that helped them achieve their goals, as well as discussed circumstances that might have been helpful for those who did not achieve their goals. Then, participants started the third module designed to promote mastery experiences. After learning about the concept of mastery and how these experiences promote recovery, participants in a small group shared the activities that helped them to experience high mastery and discussed what challenges they could engage in during leisure time.

The fourth and final module focused on relaxation and sleep. Participants engaged in a short imaginary journey to relax, before they learned about the relaxation process itself and how it could help them to recover from work. They shared the activities during which they felt relaxed and discussed common features of these activities in a group. Later, they also learned about sleep hygiene and progressive muscle relaxation techniques. Finally, participants reflected on and discussed what they already did well and what they would like to improve. Two weeks after the intervention, Hahn et al. (2011)

reported increased recovery experiences, recovery-related self-efficacy, and better sleep quality, as well as decreased stressful experience and negative affect in the intervention group, compared with a waitlist control group.

Assuming that severe job stressors are absent or weakened, recovery strategies overall are helpful for employees to replenish drained energies and depleted resources, obtain new resources, and slow down or stop further resources loss before they are back at work. Recovery experiences also counter negative effects of job stressors. Four other evidence-based organizational stress management programs are described in the following sections.

## 4.2    Improve Well-Being by Job Crafting

*Job crafting* is an employee's self-initiated job redesign behavior to change, redesign, and improve a job for themselves. Employees can proactively engage in three types of voluntary role-oriented crafting behaviors to improve their work role so that their own abilities, needs, and preferences can better align with their jobs (Wrzesniewski & Dutton, 2001). These three crafting behaviors are *task crafting* (i.e., crafting ways of performing job activities, such as seeking out additional tasks or opportunities to expand skills sets), *relational crafting* (i.e., crafting ways of interacting with others while performing job activities, such as building better relationships with experienced colleagues), and *cognitive crafting* (i.e., crafting ways of thinking about how job activities are performed, such as reframing a tedious task to be consequential). It should be emphasized that job crafting behaviors are not only about solving problems, but also about pursuing opportunities and personal growth.

Bruning and Campion (2018) expanded the conceptualization of job crafting via two dimensions: *role crafting* versus *resource crafting*, and *approach crafting* versus *avoidance crafting*. Role crafting explains people crafting their work roles to improve alignment between the requirements of their jobs and their needs and abilities. Resource crafting, drawn from the JD-R theory described in Section 2.4, explains how people acquire new resources or manage existing resources to reduce job demands and strain experiences.

Both role crafting and resource crafting behaviors can further be classified as either approach crafting activities or avoidance crafting activities. According to Bruning and Campion (2018), people who engage in approach role-based crafting activities are motivated to expand their work roles (e.g., seek out more challenges or assume more responsibilities), or expand social relationships with colleagues (e.g., increase interactions with others). In contrast, people who engage in *avoidance role-based crafting* activities actively reduce their work roles or responsibilities by giving away their tasks to others or asking others to engage in social interactions (e.g., attend a formal party) on their behalf.

When people engage in *approach resource crafting* activities, they actively increase or modify job resources to maximize their capabilities. For example, they increase job control, gain social support, or seek advice and feed-back from colleagues. They may also adopt external technologies, such as LinkedIn Learning (a subsidiary of LinkedIn that provides online video courses taught by industry experts), to improve performance. In contrast to approach resource crafting, people engage in *avoidance resource crafting* activities when they need to withdraw mentally or physically from work contexts or people (e.g., by listening to music or taking a break away from upsetting situations or people). Overall, results of two meta-analyses showed positive effects of job crafting behaviors on work engagement and job performance (Lichtenthaler & Fischbach, 2019; Rudolph et al., 2017).

There have been several successful occupational stress management interventions that train participants to apply self-initiated strategies to deal with job demands. The majority of these studies focus on ways of seeking challenges, seeking resources, and minimizing and optimizing demands (e.g., Demerouti et al., 2020; Demerouti et al., 2017; Gordon et al., 2018). A meta-analysis demonstrated positive effects of job crafting interventions on seeking challenges and reducing demands (Oprea et al., 2019). In addition, these interventions tended to improve work engagement and increase discretional behaviors to benefit organizations and others (Oprea et al., 2019).

A recent study (Kuijpers et al., 2020) focused on crafting personal strengths (i.e., making better use of one's strengths in one's work role) and interests (i.e., changing job contents to match one's interest), as well as development (i.e., creating developmental opportunities to maximize one's talents). Based on the JD-R theory (Bakker & Demerouti, 2017), Bakker and van Wingerden (2021) focused on ways of crafting personal resources (e.g., assertiveness, self-efficacy, or resilience) or ways of strengthening people's belief regarding how much control they have over their work. Box 2 is a summary of key crafting strategies based on Bakker and van Wingerden (2021), Kuijpers et al. (2020), and Demerouti et al. (2020).

In the following section, a recently developed job crafting intervention based on the JD-R theory will be described (Bakker & Demerouti, 2017). It should be noted that job crafting interventions can be applied beyond traditional occupational stress management. For instance, they have been applied to help unemployed people craft employment (Hulshof et al., 2020).

In Step 1 of a typical job crafting intervention, trainers provide training participants with concrete real-life examples of job demands, job resources, and job crafting behaviors prior to the workshop. During the workshop, training participants analyze their job demands and job resources. In a group, each participant reports one successful job crafting behavior that solved a problem at work.

In Step 2, participants are encouraged to think about how the job crafting behaviors they shared earlier may be helpful in accomplishing future goals pertaining to seeking resources and challenges, reducing job demands, and optimizing job demands. Participants also stimulate one another to discover concrete strategies to achieve future goals. This group exchange also provides an opportunity for increasing self-efficacy.

**Box 2**
**Key Crafting Strategies Applied to Job Crafting**

**Bakker & van Wingerden (2021)**

**Crafting personal resources**
- Practice openly communicating with others about desires and needs.
- Practice how to speak about feelings and how to share points of view.
- Practice how to give and receive positive and negative feedback in a respectful and constructive way.
- Practice refusing a request.
- Write reactions to recent setbacks and elaborate on different ways of framing the setbacks in constructive ways.

**Kuijpers et al. (2020)**

**Crafting personal strengths**
- Change job contents or contexts to make full use of current knowledge and capacities.
- Take on tasks that you're good at.
- Take advantage of your strengths as much as possible while performing tasks.

**Crafting interests**
- Take on tasks that you like.
- Seek out tasks that match interests.
- Organize work in such a way that you can do what you find interesting.

**Crafting development**
- Seek out opportunities to use a variety of skills at work.
- Find tasks that help develop employees.
- Identify tasks that can tap into an employee's unused knowledge and skills.

**Demerouti et al. (2020)**

**Seeking job resources**
- Ask others for feedback on job performance.
- Ask colleagues or supervisors for advice.
- Learn new things at work.
- Contact colleagues or supervisors to gather needed information for completing tasks.
- Discuss difficulties or problems at work with colleagues or supervisors.

**Seeking challenges**
- Ask for more responsibilities.
- Ask for more tasks when all regular tasks have been completed.
- Ask for more odd jobs.

**Minimizing demands**
- Ensure that work is emotionally less intense.
- Make sure that work is mentally less intense.
- Ensure that work is physically less intense.

**Optimizing demands**
- Simplify or improve work processes or procedures to make the job easier.
- Modify work processes or procedures which delay the work.
- Find ways to accomplish the work in an easier way.

In Step 3, trainers facilitate training participants to demonstrate the value of job crafting behaviors regarding increasing or managing resources, as well as reducing and optimizing job demands.

In the final step, trainers apply the goal-setting theory to encourage participants to set up four goals for the following 4 weeks after the workshop. These goals are seeking resources, optimizing demands, reducing demands, and seeking challenges. These goals direct participants' attention and energize their efforts to engage in job crafting behaviors persistently. Trainers encourage participants to identify potential factors that may facilitate or inhibit them from pursuing their goals, and think of ways to minimize obstacles and optimize facilitators in advance. In addition, trainers remind participants weekly about their goals to maintain participants' commitments to their goals. Finally, all participants share their success and failures while practicing job crafting behaviors during the program, and discuss how they could continue crafting their job after the workshop.

In sum, job crafting strategies, as summarized in Box 2 empower employees to actively take charge of redesigning their own job environment through gaining personal and job resources; pursuing personal strengths, interests, and career development; increasing job challenges; and minimizing and optimizing job demands. These strategies can be modified and applied to counter effects of job stressors or minimize or optimize job stressors themselves (e.g., role stressors, work–family conflict, workload, lack of control, organizational constraints, organizational injustice, dysfunctional organizational politics, and workplace mistreatment, etc.).

## 4.3    Supervisor as a Change Agent

In contrast to the above two types of intervention programs, the remaining intervention programs involve supervisors, either directly or indirectly. High-quality leadership has been shown in a meta-analysis to be associated with employees' mental health (Montano et al., 2017). Specifically, high-quality supervision or leadership tends to be negatively associated with subordinates' affective symptoms, burnout, job tension, job strains, and health complaints, and positively related to subordinates' well-being, empowerment, and self-worth. Furthermore, supervisors who do not stigmatize those employees with mental health problems and who possess skills that can support employees with recovery, tend to promote employees' well-being (Marchand et al., 2013). Thus, training supervisors to develop leadership skills has been considered as a bedrock upon which to build a safe and healthy workplace (Kelloway & Barling, 2010).

From both practical and theoretical perspectives, there are several advantages to focusing on training those in leadership positions. First, it is a relatively cost-effective way to combat job stressors in an organization. People in leadership positions tend to stay in organizations longer than their subordinates. In addition, behavior changes in leaders – say an increase of either positive or negative supervisor behaviors – likely have broader and lasting impacts on their subordinates' well-being and productivity. Third, emotional and instrumental supports from supervisors have shown stronger positive effects on their subordinates' well-being in a meta-analysis, compared with support from coworkers (Mathieu et al., 2019). Fourth, leaders create a climate (Lewin et al., 1939) in which employees value and respect each other, and the climate establishes norms and provides cues about how things are done and how people should or should not behave in an organization (Li et al., 2017). It is not surprising that the US Equal Employment Opportunity Commission (2016, June) recommended that the first step in creating an effective prevention program, such as a mistreatment prevention program, is putting leaders in place who are willing to shape normative values, beliefs, and behaviors in organizations so that people treat each other with respect and dignity.

### 4.3.1    Family-Supportive Supervisor Behaviors

Over the years, some organizations have developed work–family support policies to address the work–family conflict experienced by employees. Although the existence of these policies is significantly associated with a reduction of work–family conflict, as shown in at least one meta-analysis (Butts et al., 2013), the estimated effect size is relatively small (–0.08). This limitation may be improved by strengthening supervisory support (Schall & Chen, 2021). Several meta-analyses have highlighted the significant role that supervisors can play in reducing work interference with family, if they listen to subordinates' problems in this regard and help them to resolve these challenges (Kossek et al., 2011; Michel et al., 2010).

A series of intervention studies focusing on ways of increasing family-supportive supervisory behaviors have shown positive effects on physical health (Hammer et al., 2011), family relationships (Brady et al., 2021), and sleep quality and quantity (Crain et al., 2019), as well as job performance, commitment, engagement, job satisfaction, and reduced turnover intention (Odle-Dusseau et al., 2016).

According to Hammer et al. (2009), family-supportive supervisor behaviors fall into four domains: *emotional support* (i.e., express concern for subordinates' experience of work interfering with nonwork life), *instrumental support* (i.e., address subordinates' work and nonwork life needs via actions), *role modeling behaviors* (i.e., act as a role model to show subordinates how supervisors effectively manage their own work and nonwork life), and *creative work–family management* (i.e., reorganize work creatively to facilitate subordinates' performance). Family-supportive supervisor behaviors in each domain described in Hammer et al. are presented in Table 10.

One of the most recent family-supportive supervisor training programs is tied to the work of Odle-Dusseau et al. (2016). Prior to the training, subordinates of participating supervisors complete a needs assessment survey. Results of the survey assist a trainer to assess the levels of family-supportive supervisor behaviors experienced by the subordinates. In the beginning of a

**Table 10**
**Samples of Family Supportive Supervisor Behaviors**

| Support behavior | Examples |
|---|---|
| Emotional support | Empathically listen to subordinates' problems in juggling work and nonwork life. |
| | Take the time to learn about subordinates' personal needs. |
| | Make subordinates feel comfortable talking about their conflicts between work and nonwork. |
| | Talk to subordinates effectively to solve conflicts between work and nonwork issues. |
| Instrumental support | Help subordinates resolve scheduling conflicts (e.g., give them time off). |
| | Make sure subordinates' work responsibilities can be handled when they have unanticipated nonwork demands. |
| | Work with subordinates to creatively solve conflicts between work and nonwork. |
| Role model | Be a good role model for maintaining a work and nonwork balance (e.g., take a day off to meet a personal need). |
| | Demonstrate and share effective behaviors in how to juggle between work and nonwork demands. |
| | Demonstrate how a person can be successful on and off the job. |
| Creative work–family management | Think about how the work can be organized to benefit both subordinates and organizations. |
| | Ask for suggestions to make it easier for subordinates to balance work and nonwork demands. |
| | Creatively reallocate job duties to help subordinates work better as a team. |
| | Manage all subordinates as a whole team to enable everyone's needs to be met. |

Adapted from Hammer et al., 2009.

3-hr face-to-face training session, a trainer provides educational information about the individual and organizational benefits of reducing work–family conflict (e.g., well-being and job performance); ways of reducing workfamily conflict by utilizing organizational resources, such as increasing family-supportive supervisor behaviors and worklife policies; levels of family supportive supervisor behaviors perceived by participants' subordinates; and definitions and examples of the four types of family-supportive supervisor behaviors (Hammer et al., 2009).

The trainer then facilitates a series of interactive exercises. First, the trainer instructs the participants to generate examples based on their experience of a work–family dilemma faced by one of their subordinates. Then, the participants share with the group what they did in response to the dilemma. They also identify which dimensions of family-supportive behaviors their responses fall under. Following that, the trainer encourages each participant to create a list of strategies they could have utilized, by following examples of the four types of familysupportive supervisor behaviors. To motivate each participant to transfer what they have learned from the training environment back to the work environment, the trainer applies the behavioral self-monitoring principle and asks all participants to record and evaluate their family-supportive behaviors after the training. Specifically, each day over the course of 2 weeks after the training, each participant records any specific family-supportive behaviors in which they engage and submits a daily record to the trainer.

Odle-Dusseau et al. (2016) evaluated the effect of family-supportive supervisor training on subordinates' perceptions of family-supportive supervisor behaviors, organizational commitment, engagement, job satisfaction, and turnover intentions, as well as job performance as rated by their supervisors 1 month after the training. Compared with subordinates whose supervisors did not attend the training, subordinates whose supervisors received the training reported increased family-supportive supervisor behaviors, organizational commitment, engagement, job satisfaction, and job performance, and decreased turnover intentions.

### 4.3.2    Supportive Supervisor Behaviors and Job Crafting

Family-supportive supervisor training highlights a pivotal leadership role that supervisors can play while complementing the employee-initiated job crafting training described earlier. Without relying on a lot of organizational resources, supervisors can help subordinates gain personal or job resources (e.g., provide subordinates with frequent feedback), galvanize personal strengths (e.g., encourage subordinates to use their current knowledge and capacities to the fullest), develop career growth (e.g., provide subordinates with more responsibilities), minimize demands (e.g., provide subordinates with emotional and instrumental supports), and optimize demands (e.g., improve subordinates' work processes).

### 4.3.3    Improve Well-Being by Reducing Workplace Mistreatment

Mistreatment in the workplace reflects the dark side of human behavior, and it is shown in different forms, such as bullying, incivility, abusive supervision, etc. This section will focus on a workplace mistreatment prevention program that addresses often-observed mistreatment from supervisors. In addition, it will describe an approach my colleagues and I (Tuckey et al., 2015) have applied to identify risky work contexts in which workplace mistreatment tends to be perceived by employees. It has been estimated that about half of the employee population at some point in their working lifetime will experience abusive behaviors from a supervisor (Tepper & Zhou, 2017).

## Prevent Abusive Supervision by Enhancing Supportive Supervision

Keenan and Newton (1985) identified interpersonal conflict at work as one of the most frequently reported workplace mistreatments. When conflicts are not resolved, collegial social relationships at work deteriorate, and uncivil behaviors, such as rude, disrespectful, insulting, or discourteous behaviors, become more common. To reduce uncivil or abusive supervisor behaviors perceived by employees, Gonzalez-Morales et al. (2018) conducted an intervention to train supervisors to support their subordinates.

Why would supportive supervisor training reduce abusive and uncivil behaviors? Gonzalez-Morales et al. (2018) provided three theoretical reasons. First, subordinates likely reciprocate supportive supervisory behaviors via increased productivity that meets or exceeds performance goals set up by their supervisors. Hence, supervisors are less likely to engage in abusive or uncivil behaviors toward their subordinates. Second, supportive supervisors likely shape organization norms of caring, consideration, and support. As a result, these norms regulate other supervisors so that they are less likely to engage in abusive or uncivil behaviors toward their subordinates. Third, supportive supervisory behaviors are likely perceived favorably by subordinates. Hence, supportive supervisors are less likely perceived to be abusive or uncivil by their subordinates.

Prior to the intervention, Gonzalez-Morales et al. (2018) conducted a needs assessment with supervisors and subordinates in a restaurant chain. Employees were asked to list circumstances in which subordinates felt supported and unsupported, as well as incidents in which subordinates felt they were being treated positively (e.g., being treated with respect, being recognized for their efforts, etc.) or negatively (e.g., being yelled at, being unfairly disciplined, etc.).

Based on the results of the needs assessment, as well as organizational support literature, Gonzalez-Morales et al. (2018) trained supervisors to use four types of strategies to increase supportive supervisory behaviors: *benevolence*, *sincerity*, *fairness*, and *experiential processing*. The first type of strategy, benevolence, provides subordinates with emotional and instrumental support beyond the supervisor's required roles and duties. Mathieu et al. (2019) has shown in a meta-analysis that both emotional and instructional supports are negatively related to job stressors (e.g., role conflict, role ambiguity, role overload, work–family conflict), and job strains (e.g., burnout, job dissatisfaction, physical symptoms), turnover intention, and poor job performance. The second strategy, sincerity, is about showing authenticity in words and actions. The next strategy, fairness, promotes organizational justice (e.g., procedural justice, distributive justice, and interactional justice), as described in Section 3.6. Finally, the fourth strategy, experiential processing, attends to information without immediate judgment. The sample strategies described in Box 3 are modified from Gonzalez-Morales et al. (2018).

The training was conducted in four 2-hr sessions over 2 months with the first three sessions conducted in three consecutive weeks, and the fourth session, a refresher session, conducted 1 month after the third session. The training involved lectures, group discussion, and role plays based on relevant, realistic, and meaningful vignettes developed from incidents identified from the needs assessment.

---

**Box 3**
**Strategies to Increase Supportive Supervisory Behaviors**

**Benevolence**

- Recognize subordinates' efforts.
- Accept subordinates' mistakes and use their mistakes as learning opportunities to help them grow.
- Back up subordinates when necessary.
- Provide subordinates with training opportunities to do their jobs.
- Make up for poor treatment from others.

**Sincerity**

- Follow through with promises made to subordinates.
- Honestly communicate positive and negative feedback about subordinates' performances.
- Treat subordinates with respect.
- Engage in constructive feedback with subordinates by:
  - focusing on subordinates' behaviors instead of themselves
  - offering encouragement
  - recommending corrective actions
  - providing unambiguous directions and clear expectations

**Fairness**

- Procedures are developed based on accurate information.
- The same rules and policies are applied to all subordinates.
- Procedures are neutral and unbiased for all subordinates.
- Provide subordinates with opportunities to voice their concerns.
- Offer subordinates opportunities for correction or appeal.
- Be accountable for decision making and explain why decisions are made.

**Experiential Processing**

- Record and gather all relevant information regarding subordinates' performances.
- Be mindful of how, where, and when discussions with subordinates are conducted.
- Engage in active listening by:
  - avoiding interruption
  - deferring judgment
  - paying attention to what is said
  - organizing what is said
  - showing interest
  - maintaining focus on listening
  - seeking out feedback to ensure accuracy of what is said

Adapted from Gonzalez-Morales et al., 2018.

Each vignette was written to capture one or two of the strategies depicted in Box 3. For instance, a vignette described a situation in which subordinates performed poorer than expected, and the supervisors either did not provide their subordinates with immediate feedback for improvement, or reacted negatively or abusively toward their subordinates. Other examples described situations in which supervisors did not provide recognition when their subordinates performed well under challenging circumstances, or when supervisors did not apply policies consistently and played favorites with some of their subordinates.

In addition, the strategies in Box 3 were discussed in a group discussion, and group members practiced these strategies via role-playing supervisor-subordinate interactions. Role-playing members received feedback from other group members after role playing each vignette. Before the end of each training session, training participants received flashcards summarizing the strategies, and were encouraged to practice the strategies in their daily interactions with subordinates during the week after each training session. In addition, each week between training sessions, training participants reviewed examples of the strategies, recorded questions for the trainer, and documented successful and unsuccessful applications of the strategies.

Gonzalez-Morales et al. (2018) evaluated the effect of supervisor support training on subordinates' perceptions of supervisor support and abusive supervisory behaviors 9 months after the training. Compared with subordinates whose supervisors were in the control group, subordinates whose supervisors received the training reported increased perception of supervisor support and decreased abusive supervisory behaviors.

## Risk Contexts With Often-Perceived Mistreatment and Injustice

Similar to an approach used to identify high crash risk highway segments, my colleagues and I (Tuckey et al., 2015) identified five risk contexts in which workplace mistreatment and unfair treatment tend to be perceived by employees. In practice, once these risk contexts are identified, management can reduce perceived mistreatment and injustice preemptively by using the strategies described in Table 10 and Box 3, as well as strategies described in the next section.

After examining 342 mistreatment complaints lodged with SafeWork SA, Australia (similar to the US Occupational Safety and Health Administration) between 2010 and 2013, Tuckey et al. (2015) identified that 90% of mistreatment experiences fell into just five risk contexts: misuse of *human resource management* (HRM) procedures and practices, poor communication, inadequate supervision skills and actions, lack of role clarification, and inadequate performance management.

The misuse of HRM procedures involved any disputes related to finance, leave requests, or rostering and scheduling issues. A complainant stated, "The store manager and HR have a lot to answer for, constantly lying and making excuses to keep me off the work shift, no doubt hoping I'll leave." Communication was a major organizational function, and 70% of cases experienced mistreatment when the complainants interacted with their supervisors. Poor communication included having information withheld, being ignored or faced with a hostile reaction, or being excluded. For instance, a complainant wrote,

> I found that nothing I did was right. I was continually criticized or given the cold shoulder and not spoken to, information relevant to my job was not passed on to me, I was accused of not wanting my job, not knowing how to sell any more.

An example of being ignored was described by another complainant:

> After I had tried to complain about not being able to use a stool and asked for information in relation to my wages, [my manager] began to act very oddly. By this I mean that when I said good morning and progressed into 'how are you today?' she would barely speak to me and instead turned around and walked away.

Supervisory skills and actions play critical roles in building positive social relationships between supervisors and their subordinates. Inadequate supervision skills and actions often contribute to perceived mistreatment. These include having poor management skills and practices, inadequate training being provided to workers, abuse of power by managers, and favoritism, etc. A complainant wrote, "I have been receiving emails from [my manager] which were full of negative feedback. There was never any assistance in the form of coaching, mentoring or guidance from [them] on how to assist me in my position." An example of unfair treatment related to favoritism was expressed by another complainant:

> [My manager] told me he would stop my personal phone calls, and I said that in my opinion if he did that to me then it should apply to all staff members as all staff make and receive personal phone calls.... I know that everyone else in the office takes personal phone calls and I have never heard him speak to them about it.

Concerns about role clarification referred to role-related issues (e.g., role overload, role conflict, or role ambiguity) contributing to mistreatment experiences or perceptions. For instance, a complainant stated,

> Initially employed as a preschool teacher, I assisted part time on a contract for three months at [location] site. Before long, my hours and duties were increased – I felt uneasy even at this early stage as I was left with cleaning duties (including toilets, mopping and vacuuming floors) while being sole caregiver of up to 8 children.

Lodging complainants often experienced confusion regarding their responsibilities or expectations. For instance, a complaint stated that, "I have been undermined by his [the supervisor's] continued attempts to do the work normally allocated to me, causing me to fear for my job."

During formal or informal interactions regarding subordinates' performances, complainants often reported being mistreated. For instance, a complainant wrote, "[The supervisor discussed] how he would formally 'performance manage' me. I believe this was a strategy deliberately designed to break me mentally and emotionally and force me to resign long ago." Another complainant expressed how they felt they were being mistreated:

> The document I received listed a number of criteria. In part it treated me as though I had just left school while simultaneously requiring outcomes that were highly unlikely or not possible. All this was to be achieved in an unrealistic time frame. Termination was threatened if I did not meet all of the objectives.

The above risky work contexts identified from legal complaints suggest that *perceptions* of workplace mistreatment can be prevented when management uses a *work design approach* to redesign work contexts preemptively (Li et al., 2019; Tuckey et al., 2022). In other words, perceived mistreatment and injustice can be reduced or eliminated by clarifying employees' roles, strengthening organizational justice, improving performance management procedures and practices, and promoting supportive supervisory skills and actions. There were three interventions that used the work design approach to design out a risk job characteristic (i.e., lack of control) to improve employees' well-being. Principles of the work design can be adapted and applied to design out other risk characteristics or work contexts.

## 4.4   Redesigning Work to Promote Job Control

Three work design interventions were developed to increase job control, although the content of these interventions varied among the participating organizations. All three successfully developed and implemented interventions shared two common themes. First, these organization-targeted interventions had buy-in from the participating organizations. Second, these interventions were implemented with inputs from stakeholders (i.e., employees and supervisors) within the organizations at each step.

*Work design* refers to creating or modifying the contents, characteristics, structures, and contexts in which tasks are engaged and roles are enacted (Parker et al., 2017). The work design literature can be traced in numerous disciplines including medicine, industrial engineering, mechanical engineering, human factors or ergonomics, management, physiology, epidemiology, biomechanics, or psychology. Based on work design rules utilized in various disciplines, Campion and Thayer (1985) classified these rules into four approaches. The first approach, *mechanistic design*, focuses on improving performance efficiency, such as simplifying ways tasks can be economically and efficiently performed with little idle time. The second approach, *perceptual/ motor design*, takes human perceptual and motor capabilities and limitations into consideration while designing work environments and tasks to better fit with people, such as modifying lighting, arranging layouts, or reducing boredom. The third approach, *biological design*, attempts to improve workers' physical well-being by, for example, adjusting seating, modifying lifting methods, reducing repetitive motion in production, or designing tools to be used comfortably. The fourth approach, *motivational design*, aims at enriching and enhancing the motivating characteristics of a job, such as increasing an employee's sense of job control, as described in Chapter 3 (Section 3.4).

Bond and Bunce (2001) conducted a work design intervention in a government division, aiming to enhance job control. They applied a *participative action approach*, which is a collaborative process that involves stakeholders within an organization and the research team to improve initiatives undertaken. Three of six units in the divisions were assigned to the intervention and a waitlist control group, respectively. Prior to developing and implementing the intervention, 12 volunteers from three units in the intervention group were invited to serve on a steering committee which met for 2 hrs for five times over a 3-month period. Based on the results of a prior needs assessment, their experiences, and their priorities, the steering committee members proposed an action plan with strategies to improve job control over three problem areas: assignment distribution procedures, within-unit consultation and communication, and informal performance feedback. Then, the committee members shared the proposed work design strategies with members of their respective units. Each committee member facilitated discussion and revision of the proposed strategies within each unit before the final work design strategies were implemented. Twelve months after the implementation, employees from three units in the intervention group reported a significant increase in job control, mental health, and job performance, and a decrease in sickness absence, compared with members of the control group.

In a second work design intervention, Logan and Ganster (2005) conducted a brainstorming session with 14 project managers after a prior needs assessment that revealed low levels of job control experienced by project managers in a large trucking company. These project managers were encouraged to assess their jobs, identify challenges and concerns, and suggest ways to make their jobs better. After the session, the managers identified three areas that they were responsible for, over which they felt they had little control: no discretion to determine who should provide their maintenance needs (local outside vendors, shops located at the closest terminal, or either option), no discretion to help their drivers when trucks broke down after business hours, and no control to audit project profit and loss statements.

In collaboration with the maintenance department of the company, the research team developed five classes, involving a total of 10 hrs of instruction, to address each of the above three areas. Participating project managers learned how to deal with outside vendors and the terminal shops to secure truck maintenance. They were also given the discretion to make decisions regarding maintenance. The second area of concern – lack of control – was how to handle nighttime emergency road services. To address this issue, two nighttime road service dispatchers were trained to deal with emergency road services, and the participating project managers were told to contact them when nighttime road service was needed. Finally, the participating project managers learned how to audit an expense statement and how to submit requests for adjustment or correction if they found problems. Four months after the training, compared with the project managers in the control group, the project managers in the work design intervention group perceived increased control and job satisfaction. However, these positive effects were only observed for the project managers with supportive management. *The results clearly highlighted that, without buy-in and continual support from management, the benefits of work design interventions are likely attenuated.*

The third work design intervention was conducted at a call center (Holman & Axtell, 2016). During a 2-day workshop facilitated by the research team, four teams of call center agents and four team leaders in the intervention group worked in small groups to identify problems and obstacles that prevented them from performing their tasks effectively. They also discussed the pros and cons of three versions of work design: maximizing well-being, maximizing performance, and optimizing well-being and performance. Through discussing the above three scenarios, participants were asked to propose changes that would optimize well-being and performance. Suggested changes were then rated, based on their overall effects. At the end of the workshop, participants were asked to develop workable proposals within 2 weeks for each proposed change.

These proposals were then discussed by participants (i.e., call center agents and their team leaders), management, and the research team at a meeting. Five major changes were proposed, including giving agents discretion over when to complete team administrative tasks, giving agents discretion over complaint handling, improving clarity with regard to the criteria used to assess agents' job performance, offering agents training on how to handle complaints, and giving agents responsibility for running weekly team briefings. These implementations were expected to enhance job control as well as feedback about agents' performance.

During the 4-month implementation phase, agents and the team leaders of each team were tasked with implementing the proposed changes described above. They also monitored if the changes worked and provided improvements. The research team also attended all team meetings to discuss progress and raise questions with management if any of the teams encountered difficulty with implementation.

Approximately 2 to 3 months after the implementation, results showed an improvement in agents' job control, well-being, and job performance, as well as an increase in receiving feedback about their performance, compared with agents in the control group.

## 4.5    A Final Note

Given that health professionals face diverse job stressors that occur in a variety of organizations and occupations, how can we successfully apply the preventive organizational stress management interventions described in this chapter? Indeed, it may seem a daunting task to address different job stressors occurring in different organizations. Past research (e.g., Day & Penney, 2019; Nielsen et al., 2010) has provided practical recommendations to assist health professionals when they are asked to assist organizations to prevent or reduce job stressors. These recommendations can be summarized as three essential elements to ensure successful interventions, which are described below.

All of the intervention programs described in this chapter (i.e., improving recovery experiences, enhancing job crafting behaviors, improving supportive supervisor behaviors to reduce work–family conflict, preventing workplace mistreatment, and redesigning work to increase job control) were sponsored by participating organizations. Thus, the first and the most important element to ensure successful interventions is to *gain buy-in from organizations and support from most of the management teams before developing and implementing organizational stress management interventions.*

While consulting with organizations regarding occupational stress issues, I have often heard from some management team members who believe that exposure to job stressors is inevitable. These managers often do not believe it is an urgent concern from the employees' perspectives, because employees are only concerned about their paycheck. Once, a senior executive officer of a state government agency declined to participate in a federally funded violence prevention project, even though her HR director enthusiastically supported the project, due to recent fatalities attributed to workplace violence. Her rationale was that her agency would be liable if the agency did not act on any recommendations derived from the proposed project. My personal experiences, however, are not unique. Pfeffer et al. (2020) interviewed 21 executives from 20 progressive companies. Although most of the executives felt that they were responsible for the well-being of employees and their families (but not for temporary or contract workers), they were reluctant to rethink work design, were unwilling to invest in employees who were likely to leave, and viewed the work and the work environment as unchangeable. Philosophically, they believed that a healthy workforce is a means to an end, rather than viewing employees' well-being as an end in itself. The rigid beliefs held by these progressive executives illustrate the stiff challenges involved in eliminating or minimizing job stressors in the majority of organizations.

Once buy-in from the organization and most management team members is ensured, the second essential element to ensure successful interventions is to *empower stakeholders* (i.e., employees and their supervisors) *to be involved at each stage of initiatives.* Applying a participative action approach, management team and health professionals can empower employees and their supervisors to identify and monitor job stressors via needs assessment (e.g., qualitative and quantitative assessment) so that it becomes clear that change is necessary. Based on the needs assessment results, the management team can communicate clearly with employees and their supervisors that they support the initiatives.

My colleagues and I (Wiegand et al., 2012), participating in a US National Institute for Occupational Safety and Health panel, have identified a list of job stressors, such as role stressors, workload, job control, organizational constraints, organizational injustice, or mistreatments, which are both *malleable* (i.e., these job stressors can be relatively easy to change or control), and *actionable* (i.e., organizations can reasonably intervene). Sources of self-report assessment tools can be found in Appendix 3. These tools can also be complemented with interviewing stakeholders, brainstorming with stakeholders, auditing existing operational procedures, and reviewing work contexts and contents via O*NET.

After identifying key job stressors, the third essential element to ensure successful interventions is that the management team, stakeholders, and health professionals *work together to modify and tailor evidence-based occupational stress management programs* to meet their needs, before implementing the intervention. Furthermore, stakeholders should be involved in assessing whether or not the intervention meets planned goals. To motivate stakeholders to sustain and institutionalize these initiatives after health professionals leave, it is helpful for them to know what works, what does not work, what obstacles there are, and what to do about these obstacles when these initiatives do not work.

Occupational safety and health research has consistently pointed out that management commitment plays a vital role to manage safety and health concerns (e.g., Pfeffer et al., 2020; Schall & Chen, 2021). The commitment and subsequent change initiatives are primarily driven by business urgency (Kotter, 1995). To ensure successful occupational stress management initiatives, it is important for management to develop a sense of urgency about psychosocial risks at work as well as their adverse impacts on employees and organizations, communicate the urgency broadly with key constituencies, prioritize resources to minimize psychosocial risks, and institutionalize preventive strategies.

# 5

# Case Vignette

Melinda and her team members have been leading the product development department at an E-commerce company. They recently experienced mass layoffs in their organization. Although her team was not affected by the change, her team members and she have experienced high levels of anxiety because of job insecurity.

In addition, her team members have complained to her about the high volume of work they were asked to do to cover human resource shortages. It has been challenging for her team members and her to complete daunting tasks within a limited time. She observed frustration, irritation, and low energy among the team at work.

One of her team members, Isabel, told her lately that she had felt emotionally exhausted and worn-out after long hours of work. She could not fall asleep easily and often woke up several times each night. Isabel was also not able to distance herself from the work, or relax and enjoy leisure time with her family.

Another team member, Hollie, had been in a sad and anxious mood after work, yet constantly thought about work when she was with her significant other. Hollie also expressed her life was far from ideal.

Melinda also had similar feelings and had experienced a lack of confidence in herself. At a recent leadership meeting, other managers also expressed similar concerns for their unit members who have shown physical or psychological strains.

## Organizational Diagnosis

The leadership team sought assistance from a professional consulting firm that specializes in enhancing workplace wellbeing. Based on the initial interview with several employees and unit leaders, a consultant conducted a needs assessment to identify to what extent employees could unwind after their work. After implementing the Recovery Experience Questionnaire (see Appendix 2; Sonnentag & Fritz, 2007), the consultant found that the majority of employees could not mentally distance themselves from work and disengage from work-related activities in the evenings and during the weekends. Furthermore, some of them were unable to determine when and how to spend their leisure time, or to engage in off-work activities that met their needs. The results also revealed they had a hard time relaxing to replenish mental and physical energies drained from time pressure at work. Overall, they could not mentally switch off job-related activities, had difficulty in unwinding work pressures, and constantly had negative thoughts about their work and worrying things beyond their control.

## Recommended Intervention Strategies

Based on the results of needs assessment, the consultant recommended that the organization consider ways of improving employees' recovery from work. Specifically, the consultant suggested strengthening employees' ability to physically or mentally distance and disengage themselves from their jobs (i.e., detachment from work). Employees who could not detach from work tend to be occupied by work duties during their leisure time, think about work-related problems or challenges in the presence of their family members or friends, and become less engaged at work due to depleted energy. Past research has shown sleep problems, emotional exhaustion, health complaints, emotional instability, disengagement at work, and negative work-related thinking increase when employees fail to detach themselves from work during their leisure time.

The consultant recommended employees via an in-house training to practice the following strategies to strengthen their ability to detach from work during their leisure time. Positive intervention results are reported in Section 4.1.

- Set up an off-work schedule and expectations in advance for off-job hours (e.g., no email/voice mail contact),
- Use skills and availability of other people to help maintain work and home boundary.
- Use technology to create boundaries between work and home domain.
- Erect physical borders or physical distance between work and nonwork domains, and triage and prioritize urgent and important work and home demands.
- Separate work artifacts (e.g., office materials, office photos) from home artifacts (e.g., home materials, family/friend photos).
- Spend leisure time on activities that best fit each individual's preferences. For instance, getting away from home and visiting a remote area.
- Engage in physical activities (dancing, jogging, swimming, exercise, yoga, walking), and practice muscle relaxation, meditation, or mindfulness during leisure time or lunch breaks at work.
- Socialize with friends while at the same time reducing social demands (e.g., attending formal parties) during leisure time if needed.
- Use Ellis's (1977) ABC thought awareness exercise to regulate emotions. Reduce emotional responses toward a stressful event by changing the appraisal of the event (e.g., reappraise the situation or consider resources available to deal with the event).

- Reduce emotional responses toward a stressful event by using attentional deployment (i.e., shifting attention to positive and enjoyable events).
- Reduce job demands via problem-solving.
- Reduce job demands through self-initiated work design (e.g., job crafting).
- Increase resources through self-initiated work design.
- Practice sleep hygiene to improve sleep.
- Engage in positive work reflection (e.g., write down three good job-related events that happened at work that day and explain why these positive events occurred).
- Reduce rumination via adopting different perspectives, practicing mindfulness (e.g., a combination of meditation, total body awareness, yoga, etc.), practicing distraction (e.g., purposely focus on positive events or activities such as watching a movie), or reappraising situations or sources of job strains (e.g., view it as a personal challenge or opportunity to grow).
- Take work breaks regularly during workdays.

# 6

# Further Reading

Brown, K. G., & Gerhardt, M. W. (2002). Formative evaluation: An integrative practice model and case study. *Personnel Psychology, 55,* 951–983. https://doi.org/10.1111/j.1744-6570.2002.tb00137.x
To address the complexity of intervention programs, this article describes how to assess effectiveness of interventions during design and development, beyond focusing on outcomes.

Burke, R. J., & Richardsen, A. M. (Eds.). (2019). *Creating psychologically healthy workplaces.* Edward Elgar.
A comprehensive edited book that addresses several key topics, including what constitutes psychologically (un)healthy workplaces, ways of strengthening employees' resources, and promoting happiness, as well as organizational-level initiatives to create a psychologically healthy workplace, to support caregiving responsibilities, and to create aging-friendly workplaces.

Kidd, S. A., & Kral, M. J. (2005). Practicing participatory action research. *Journal of Counseling Psychology, 52,* 187–195. https://doi.org/10.1037/0022-0167.52.2.187
This article points out that the attitude of professionals is the key in the process of developing and implementing a successful initiative. It further encourages us to be vigilant in examining our own motives, beliefs, values, and roles, when we are called upon to assist employees and organizations.

Hobfoll, S. E., Halbesleben, J., Neveu, J. P., & Westman, M. (2018). Conservation of resources in the organizational context: The reality of resources and their consequences. *Annual Review of Organizational Psychology and Organizational Behavior, 5,* 103–128. https://doi.org/10.1146/annurev-orgpsych-032117-104640
This article reviews conservation of resources (COR) theory, which is partially the basis of job demands–resources theory. Although it is not an occupational stress theory per se, COR theory suggests that the threat of losing resources can be stressful, and we are motivated to maintain and/or gain resources. The article details basic principles and propositions of the COR theory, and suggests resources that can be built up at work for employees.

Noe, R. A., & Kodwani, A. D. (2018). *Employee training and development* (7th ed.). McGraw-Hill Education.
This book introduces key elements of training or intervention design, how to determine intervention needs, how employees learn and transfer training, and how to create an environment conducive to intervention programs.

# 7

# References

Abramis, D. J. (1994). Work role ambiguity, job satisfaction, and job performance: Meta-analyses and review. *Psychological Reports, 75,* 1411–1433. https://doi.org/10.2466/pr0.1994.75.3f.1411

Alarcon, G. M. (2011). A meta-analysis of burnout with job demands, resources, and attitudes. *Journal of Vocational Behavior, 79,* 549–562. https://doi.org/10.1016/j.jvb.2011.03.007

Allen, N. J., & Meyer, J. P. (1996). Affective, continuance, and normative commitment to the organization: An examination of construct validity. *Journal of Vocational Behavior, 49,* 252–276. https://doi.org/10.1006/jvbe.1996.0043

American Psychiatric Association. (2013). *Diagnostic and statistical manual of mental disorders* (5th ed.).

American Psychological Association. (2019). *Stress in America™ 2019.* https://www.apa.org/news/press/releases/stress/2019/stress-america-2019.pdf

Amstad, F. T., Meier, L. L., Fasel, U., Elfering, A., & Semmer, N. K. (2011). A meta-analysis of work–family conflict and various outcomes with a special emphasis on cross-domain versus matching-domain relations. *Journal of Occupational Health Psychology, 16,* 151–169. https://doi.org/10.1037/a0022170

Associated Press. (2021, February 12). *Amazon faces biggest union push in its history.* https://apnews.com/article/amazon-workers-union-c8493c24dabe7609de8fec8716460737

Bakker, A. B., & Demerouti, E. (2014). Job Demands-Resources theory. In P. Y. Chen & C. L. Cooper (Eds.), *Wellbeing: A complete reference guide, work and wellbeing* (Vol. 3; pp. 37–64). John Wiley.

Bakker, A. B., & Demerouti, E. (2017). Job demands–resources theory: Taking stock and looking forward. *Journal of Occupational Health Psychology, 22,* 273–285. https://doi.org/10.1037/ocp0000056

Bakker, A. B., & van Wingerden, J. (2021). Do personal resources and strengths use increase work engagement? The effects of a training intervention. *Journal of Occupational Health Psychology, 26,* 20–30. https://doi.org/10.1037/ocp0000266

Barber, L. K., & Santuzzi, A. M. (2015). Please respond ASAP: Workplace telepressure and employee recovery. *Journal of Occupational Health Psychology, 20,* 172–189. https://doi.org/10.1037/a0038278

Bandura, A. (1991). Social cognitive theory of self-regulation. *Organizational Behavior and Human Decision Processes, 50,* 248–287. https://doi.org/10.1016/0749-5978(91)90022-L

Bartlett, L., Martin, A., Neil, A. L., Memish, K., Otahal, P., Kilpatrick, M., & Sanderson, K. (2019). A systematic review and meta-analysis of workplace mindfulness training randomized controlled trials. *Journal of Occupational Health Psychology, 24,* 108–126. https://doi.org/10.1037/ocp0000146

BBC. (2020, January 17,). *How the Japanese are putting an end to extreme work weeks.* https://www.bbc.com/worklife/article/20200114-how-the-japanese-are-putting-an-end-to-death-from-overwork

Beehr, T. A., Bowling, N. A., & Bennett, M. M. (2010). Occupational stress and failures of social support: When helping hurts. *Journal of Occupational Health Psychology, 15,* 45–59. https://doi.org/10.1037/a0018234

Beehr, T. A., & Newman, J. E. (1978). Job stress, employee health, and organizational effectiveness: A facet analysis, model, and literature review. *Personnel Psychology, 31*, 665–699. https://doi.org/10.1111/j.1744-6570.1978.tb02118.x

Bellarosa, C., & Chen, P. Y. (1997). The effectiveness and practicality of occupational stress management interventions: A survey of subject matter expert opinions. *Journal of Occupational Health Psychology, 2*, 247–262. https://doi.org/10.1037/1076-8998.2.3.247

Bennett, A. A., Bakker, A. B., & Field, J. G. (2018). Recovery from work-related effort: A meta-analysis. *Journal of Organizational Behavior, 39*, 262–275. https://doi.org/10.1002/job.2217

Bliese, P. D., Edwards, J. R., & Sonnentag, S. (2017). Stress and well-being at work: A century of empirical trends reflecting theoretical and societal influences. *Journal of Applied Psychology, 102*, 389–402. https://doi.org/10.1037/apl0000109

Bond, F. W., & Bunce, D. (2001). Job control mediates change in a work reorganization intervention for stress reduction. *Journal of Occupational Health Psychology, 6*, 290–302. https://doi.org/10.1037/1076-8998.6.4.290

Bowling, N. A., Alarcon, G. M., Bragg, C. B., & Hartman, M. J. (2015). A meta-analytic examination of the potential correlates and consequences of workload. *Work & Stress, 29*, 95–113. https://doi.org/10.1080/02678373.2015.1033037

Bowling, N. A., & Beehr, T. A. (2006). Workplace harassment from the victim's perspective: A theoretical model and meta-analysis. *Journal of Applied Psychology, 91*, 998–1012. https://doi.org/10.1037/0021-9010.91.5.998

Brady, J. M., Hammer, L. B., Mohr, C. D., & Bodner, T. E. (2021). Supportive supervisor training improves family relationships among employee and spouse dyads. *Journal of Occupational Health Psychology, 26*, 31–48. https://doi.org/10.1037/ocp0000264

Brodie's Law. (2011). https://www.justice.vic.gov.au/safer-communities/crime-prevention/bullying-brodies-law

Bruning, P. F., & Campion, M. A. (2018). A role-resource approach-avoidance model of job crafting: A multimethod integration and extension of job crafting theory. *Academy of Management Journal, 61*, 499–522. https://doi.org/10.5465/amj.2015.0604

Burke, R. J. (2019). Creating psychologically healthy workplaces. In R. J. Burke & A. M. Richardsen (Eds.), *Creating psychologically healthy workplaces* (pp. 2–41). Edward Elgar. https://doi.org/10.4337/9781788113427.00008

Butts, M. M., Casper, W. J., & Yang, T. S. (2013). How important are work–family support policies? A meta-analytic investigation of their effects on employee outcomes. *Journal of Applied Psychology, 98*, 1–25. https://doi.org/10.1037/a0030389

Campion, M. A., & Thayer, P. W. (1985). Development and field evaluation of an interdisciplinary measure of job design. *Journal of Applied Psychology, 70*, 29–43. https://doi.org/10.1037/0021-9010.70.1.29

Cangiano, F., Parker, S. K., & Ouyang, K. (2021). Too proactive to switch off: When taking charge drains resources and impairs detachment. *Journal of Occupational Health Psychology, 26*, 142–154. https://doi.org/10.1037/ocp0000265

Caplan, R. D. (1987). Person-environment fit theory and organizations: Commensurate dimensions, time perspectives, and mechanisms. *Journal of Vocational Behavior, 31*, 248–267. https://doi.org/10.1016/0001-8791(87)90042-X

Carlson, D. S., Kacmar, K. M., & Williams, L. J. (2000). Construction and initial validation of a multidimensional measure of work-family conflict. *Journal of Vocational Behavior, 56*, 249–276. https://doi.org/10.1006/jvbe.1999.1713

Carver, C. S., Scheier, M. F., & Weintraub, J. K. (1989). Assessing coping strategies: a theoretically based approach. *Journal of Personality and Social Psychology, 56*, 267–283. https://doi.org/10.1037/0022-3514.56.2.267

Chang, C. H., Rosen, C. C., & Levy, P. E. (2009). The relationship between perceptions of organizational politics and employee attitudes, strain, and behavior: A meta-analytic examination. *Academy of Management Journal, 52*, 779–801. https://doi.org/10.5465/amj.2009.43670894

Chen, P. Y. (1991). *Effects of objective job stressors, job satisfaction, negative mood, and negative affectivity on perceived job conditions* [Unpublished doctoral dissertation]. University of South Florida.

Chen, P. Y., Li, Y., & Wu, H. (2023). Impacts of stress and well-being on organizations and societies: A global perspective. In L. M. Lapierre & C. Cooper (Eds.), *Cambridge companion to organisational stress and well-being.* Cambridge University Press. https://doi.org/10.1017/9781009268332.004

Chiou, S. S., Pan, C. S., & Keane, P. (2000). *Traumatic injury among drywall installers,* 1992 to 1995. *Journal of Occupational and Environmental Medicine, 42,* 1101-1108. https://doi.org/10.1097/00043764-200011000-00013

Cohen, J. (1988). *Statistical power analysis for the behavioral sciences* (2nd ed.). Lawrence Erlbaum Associates.

Cohen, S., Tyrrell, D. A., & Smith, A. P. (1991). Psychological stress and susceptibility to the common cold. *New England Journal of Medicine, 325,* 606-612. https://doi.org/10.1056/NEJM199108293250903

Cohen-Charash, Y., & Spector, P. E. (2001). The role of justice in organizations: A meta-analysis. *Organizational Behavior and Human Decision Processes, 86,* 278-321. https://doi.org/10.1016/S0749-5978(02)00040-7

Colquitt, J. A., Conlon, D. E., Wesson, M. J., Porter, C. O. L. H., & Ng, K. Y. (2001). Justice at the millennium: A meta-analytic review of 25 years of organizational justice research. *Journal of Applied Psychology, 86,* 425-445. https://doi.org/10.1037/0021-9010.86.3.425

Cores, S. E., Sayed, A., Tracy, D. K., & Kempton, M. J. (2021). Individual-focused Occupational Health Interventions: A meta-analysis of randomized controlled trials. *Journal of Occupational Health Psychology, 26,* 189-203. https://doi.org/10.1037/ocp0000249

Crain, T. L., Hammer, L. B., Bodner, T., Olson, R., Kossek, E. E., Moen, P., & Buxton, O. M. (2019). Sustaining sleep: Results from the randomized controlled work, family, and health study. *Journal of Occupational Health Psychology, 24,* 180-197. https://doi.org/10.1037/ocp0000122

Crawford, E. R., LePine, J. A., & Rich, B. L. (2010). Linking job demands and resources to employee engagement and burnout: A theoretical extension and meta-analytic test. *Journal of Applied Psychology, 95,* 834-848. https://doi.org/10.1037/a0019364

Cropanzano, R., Prehar, C. A., & Chen, P. Y. (2002). Using social exchange theory to distinguish procedural from interactional justice. *Group & Organization Management, 27,* 324-351. https://doi.org/10.1177/1059601102027003002

Cropanzano, R., & Wright, T. A. (2011). The impact of organizational justice on occupational health. In J. C. Quick & L. E. Tetrick (Eds.), *Handbook of occupational health psychology* (2nd ed., pp. 205-219). American Psychological Association.

Day, A., & Penney, S. A. (2019). Essential elements of organizational initiatives to improve workplace wellbeing. In R. J. Burke & A. M. Richardsen (Eds.), *Creating psychologically healthy workplaces* (pp. 314-331). Edward Elgar.

Demerouti, E., Bakker, A. B., Nachreiner, F., & Schaufeli, W. B. (2001). The job demands-resources model of burnout. *Journal of Applied Psychology, 86,* 499-512. https://doi.org/10.1037/0021-9010.86.3.499

Demerouti, E., Soyer, L. M., Vakola, M., & Xanthopoulou, D. (2020). The effects of a job crafting intervention on the success of an organizational change effort in a blue-collar work environment. *Journal of Occupational and Organizational Psychology, 94,* 374-399. https://doi.org/10.1111/joop.12330

Demerouti, E., Xanthopoulou, D., Petrou, P., & Karagkounis, C. (2017). Does job crafting assist dealing with organizational changes due to austerity measures? Two studies among Greek employees. *European Journal of Work and Organizational Psychology, 26,* 574-589. https://doi.org/10.1080/1359432X.2017.1325875

Descatha, A., Sembajwe, G., Pega, F., Ujita, Y., Baer, M., Boccuni, F., Teccoi, C. D., Duret, C., Evanoff, B. A., Gagliardi, D., Godderis, L., Kang, S. K., Kim, B. J., Li, J., Hanson, L. L. M., Marinaccio, A., Ozguler, A., Pachito, D., Pell, J., ... Iavicoli, S.

(2021). The effect of exposure to long working hours on stroke: A systematic review and meta-analysis from the WHO/ILO joint estimates of the work-related burden of disease and injury. *Environment International, 142.* https://doi.org/10.1016/j.envint.2021.106595

Eatough, E. M., Chang, C. H., Miloslavic, S. A., & Johnson, R. E. (2011). Relationships of role stressors with organizational citizenship behavior: A meta-analysis. *Journal of Applied Psychology, 96,* 619–632. https://doi.org/10.1037/a0021887

Edwards, J. R., & Cooper, C. L. (1990). The person-environment fit approach to stress: Recurring problems and some suggested solutions. *Journal Of Organizational Behavior, 11,* 293–307. https://doi.org/10.1002/job.4030110405

Ellis, A. (1977). The basic clinical theory of rational-emotive therapy. In A. Ellis & R. E. Grieger (Eds.), *Handbook of rational-emotive therapy* (pp. 3–34). Springer.

European Agency for Safety and Health at Work. (2018). *Management of psychosocial risks in European workplaces – Evidence from the second European survey of enterprises on new and emerging risks.* https://osha.europa.eu/en/publications/management-psychosocial-risks-european-workplaces-evidence-second-european-survey

Ferris, G. R., & Kacmar, K. M. (1992). Perceptions of organizational politics. *Journal of Management, 18,* 93–116. https://doi.org/10.1177/014920639201800107

Folkman, S., Lazarus, R. S., Dunkel-Schetter, C., DeLongis, A., & Gruen, R. J. (1986). Dynamics of a stressful encounter: Cognitive appraisal, coping, and encounter outcomes. *Journal of Personality and Social Psychology, 50,* 992–1003. https://doi.org/10.1037/0022-3514.50.5.992

Frese, M., & Zapf, D. (1994). Action as the core of work psychology: A German approach. In H. C. Triandis, M. D. Dunnette, & L. M. Hough (Eds.), *Handbook of industrial and organizational psychology* (2nd ed., Vol. 4, pp. 271–340). Consulting Psychologists Press.

Ganster, D. C. (1989). Worker control and well-being: A review of research in the workplace. In S. L. Sauter, J. J. Hurrell, & C. L. Cooper (Eds.), *Job control and worker health* (pp. 3–24). Wiley.

Ganster, D. C., Crain, T. L., & Brossoit, R. M. (2018). Physiological measurement in the organizational sciences: A review and recommendations for future use. *Annual Review of Organizational Psychology and Organizational Behavior, 5,* 267–293. https://doi.org/10.1146/annurev-orgpsych-032117-104613

Ganster, D. C., Fox, M. L., & Dwyer, D. J. (2001). Explaining employees' health care costs: A prospective examination of stressful job demands, personal control, and physiological reactivity. *Journal of Applied Psychology, 86,* 954–964. https://doi.org/10.1037/0021-9010.86.5.954

Gilboa, S., Shirom, A., Fried, Y., & Cooper, C. (2008). A meta-analysis of work demand stressors and job performance: Examining main and moderating effects. *Personnel Psychology, 61,* 227–271. https://doi.org/10.1111/j.1744-6570.2008.00113.x

Goh, J., Pfefer, J., & Zenios, S. A. (2015). Workplace stressors & health outcomes: Health policy for the workplace. *Behavioral Science & Policy, 1,* 43–52. https://doi.org/10.1353/bsp.2015.0001

Goh, J., Pfeffer, J., & Zenios, S. A. (2016). The relationship between workplace stressors and mortality and health costs in the United States. *Management Science, 62,* 608–628. https://doi.org/10.1287/mnsc.2014.2115

Gonzalez-Morales, M. G., Kernan, M. C., Becker, T. E., & Eisenberger, R. (2018). Defeating abusive supervision: Training supervisors to support subordinates. *Journal of Occupational Health Psychology, 23,* 151–162. https://doi.org/10.1037/ocp0000061

Gonzalez-Mulé, E., Kim, M. (M.), & Ryu, J. W. (2021). A meta-analytic test of multiplicative and additive models of job demands, resources, and stress. *Journal of Applied Psychology, 106,* 1391–1411. https://doi.org/10.1037/apl0000840

Gordon, H. J., Demerouti, E., Le Blanc, P. M., Bakker, A. B., Bipp, T., & Verhagen, M. A. M. T. (2018). Individual job redesign: Job crafting interventions in healthcare. *Journal of Vocational Behavior, 104,* 98–114. https://doi.org/10.1016/j.jvb.2017.07.002

Grandey, A. A., & Melloy, R. C. (2017). The state of the heart: Emotional labor as emotion regulation reviewed and revised. *Journal of Occupational Health Psychology, 22,* 407–422. https://doi.org/10.1037/ocp0000067

Gray, C. E., Spector, P. E., Lacey, K. N., Young, B. G., Jacobsen, S. T., & Taylor, M. R. (2020). Helping may be harming: Unintended negative consequences of providing social support. *Work & Stress, 34,* 359–385. https://doi.org/10.1080/02678373.2019.1695294

Greenberg, J. (2010). Organizational injustice as an occupational health risk. *Academy of Management Annals, 4,* 205–243. https://doi.org/10.5465/19416520.2010.481174

Greenhaus, J. H., & Beutell, N. J. (1985). Sources of conflict between work and family roles. *Academy of Management Review, 10,* 76–88. https://doi.org/10.5465/amr.1985.4277352

Grinza, E., & Rycx, F. (2020). The impact of sickness absenteeism on firm productivity: New evidence from Belgian matched employer–employee panel data. *Industrial Relations, 59,* 150–194. https://doi.org/10.1111/irel.12252

Guthier, C., Dormann, C., & Voelkle, M. C. (2020). Reciprocal effects between job stressors and burnout: A continuous time meta-analysis of longitudinal studies. *Psychological Bulletin, 146,* 1146–1173. https://doi.org/10.1037/bul0000304

Hackman, J. R., & Oldham, G. R. (1976). Motivation through the design of work: Test of a theory. *Organizational behavior and human performance, 16,* 250–279. https://doi.org/10.1016/0030-5073(76)90016-7

Hahn, V. C., Binnewies, C., Sonnentag, S., & Mojza, E. J. (2011). Learning how to recover from job stress: Effects of a recovery training program on recovery, recovery-related self-efficacy, and well-being. *Journal of Occupational Health Psychology, 16,* 202–216. https://doi.org/10.1037/a0022169

Hammer, L. B., Kossek, E. E., Anger, W. K., Bodner, T., & Zimmerman, K. L. (2011). Clarifying work-family intervention processes: The roles of work-family conflict and family-supportive supervisor behaviors. *Journal of Applied Psychology, 96,* 134–150. https://doi.org/10.1037/a0020927

Hammer, L. B., Kossek, E. E., Yragui, N. L., Bodner, T. E., & Hanson, G. C. (2009). Development and validation of a multidimensional measure of family supportive supervisor behaviors (FSSB). *Journal of Management, 35,* 837–856. https://doi.org/10.1177/0149206308328510

Hassard, J., Teoh, K. R., & Cox, T. (2019). Estimating the economic burden posed by work-related violence to society: A systematic review of cost-of-illness studies. *Safety Science, 116,* 208–221. https://doi.org/10.1016/j.ssci.2019.03.013

Hassard, J., Teoh, K. R., Visockaite, G., Dewe, P., & Cox, T. (2018a). The cost of work-related stress to society: A systematic review. *Journal of Occupational Health Psychology, 23,* 1–17. https://doi.org/10.1037/ocp0000069

Hassard, J., Teoh, K. R., Visockaite, G., Dewe, P., & Cox, T. (2018b). The financial burden of psychosocial workplace aggression: A systematic review of cost-of-illness studies. *Work & Stress, 32,* 6–32. https://doi.org/10.1080/02678373.2017.1380726

Hershcovis, M. S. (2011). "Incivility, social undermining, bullying...Oh My!": A call to reconcile constructs within workplace aggression research. *Journal of Organizational Behavior, 32,* 499–519. https://doi.org/10.1002/job.689

Hershcovis, M. S., Turner, N., Barling, J., Arnold, K. A., Dupré, K. E., Inness, M., LeBlanc, M. M., & Sivanathan, N. (2007). Predicting workplace aggression: A meta-analysis. *Journal of Applied Psychology, 92,* 228–238. https://doi.org/10.1037/0021-9010.92.1.228

Holman, D., & Axtell, C. (2016). Can job redesign interventions influence a broad range of employee outcomes by changing multiple job characteristics? A quasi-experimental study. *Journal of Occupational Health Psychology, 21,* 284–295. https://doi.org/10.1037/a0039962

Horan, K. A., Nakahara, W. H., DiStaso, M. J., & Jex, S. M. (2020). A review of the challenge-hindrance stress model: Recent advances, expanded paradigms, and recommendations for future research. *Frontiers in Psychology, 11,* 560346. https://doi.org/10.3389/fpsyg.2020.560346

Howard, M. C., Cogswell, J. E., & Smith, M. B. (2020). The antecedents and outcomes of workplace ostracism: A meta-analysis. *Journal of Applied Psychology, 105,* 577–596. https://doi.org/10.1037/apl0000453

Hülsheger, U. R., Lang, J. W., Schewe, A. F., & Zijlstra, F. R. (2015). When regulating emotions at work pays off: A diary and an intervention study on emotion regulation and customer tips in service jobs. *Journal of Applied Psychology, 100,* 263–277. https://doi.org/10.1037/a0038229

Hülsheger, U. R., & Schewe, A. F. (2011). On the costs and benefits of emotional labor: A meta-analysis of three decades of research. *Journal of Occupational Health Psychology, 16,* 361–389. https://doi.org/10.1037/a0022876

Hulshof, I. L., Demerouti, E., & Le Blanc, P. M. (2020). A job search demands-resources intervention among the unemployed: Effects on well-being, job search behavior and reemployment chances. *Journal of Occupational Health Psychology, 25,* 17–31. https://doi.org/10.1037/ocp0000167

Ilies, R., Huth, M., Ryan, A. M., & Dimotakis, N. (2015). Explaining the links between workload, distress, and work–family conflict among school employees: Physical, cognitive, and emotional fatigue. *Journal of Educational Psychology, 107,* 1136–1149. https://doi.org/10.1037/edu0000029

International Labour Organization. (2016). *Workplace stress: A collective challenge.* https://www.ilo.org/safework/info/publications/WCMS_466547/lang--en/index.htm

Jackson, S. E., & Schuler, R. S. (1985). A meta-analysis and conceptual critique of research on role ambiguity and role conflict in work settings. *Organizational Behavior and Human Decision Processes, 36,* 16–78. https://doi.org/10.1016/0749-5978(85)90020-2

Japan Times. (2019). *Subaru death-from-overwork probe finds 3,400 staff were not paid overtime for two years.* https://www.japantimes.co.jp/news/2019/01/25/business/corporate-business/subaru-death-overwork-probe-finds-3400-staff-not-paid-overtime-two-years/

Jex, S. M., Beehr, T. A., & Roberts, C. K. (1992). The meaning of occupational stress items to survey respondents. *Journal of Applied Psychology, 77,* 623–628. https://doi.org/10.1037/0021-9010.77.5.623

Johnson, J. V., & Hall, E. M. (1988). Job strain, work place social support, and cardiovascular disease: A cross-sectional study of a random sample of the Swedish working population. *American Journal of Public Health, 78,* 1336–1342. https://doi.org/10.2105/AJPH.78.10.1336

Joyce, S., Shand, F., Tighe, J., Laurent, S. J., Bryant, R. A., & Harvey, S. B. (2018). Road to resilience: A systematic review and meta-analysis of resilience training programmes and interventions. *BMJ Open, 8,* e017858. https://doi.org/10.1136/bmjopen-2017-017858

Kahn, R. L., Wolfe, D. M., Quinn, R. P., Snoek, J. D., & Rosenthal, R. A. (1964). *Organizational stress: Studies in role conflict and ambiguity.* Wiley.

Karabinski, T., Haun, V. C., Nübold, A., Wendsche, J., & Wegge, J. (2021). Interventions for improving psychological detachment from work: A meta-analysis. *Journal of Occupational Health Psychology, 26,* 224–242. https://doi.org/10.1037/ocp0000280

Karasek Jr, R. A. (1979). Job demands, job decision latitude, and mental strain: Implications for job redesign. *Administrative Science Quarterly, 24*(2), 285–308. https://doi.org/10.2307/2392498

Keenan, A., & Newton, T. J. (1985). Stressful events, stressors, and psychological strains in young professional engineers. *Journal of Occupational Behavior, 6,* 151–156. https://www.jstor.org/stable/3000249 https://doi.org/10.1002/job.4030060206

Kelloway, E. K., & Barling, J. (2010). Leadership development as an intervention in occupational health psychology. *Work & Stress, 24,* 260–279. https://doi.org/10.1080/02678373.2010.518441

Kossek, E. E., Pichler, S., Bodner, T., & Hammer, L. B. (2011). Workplace social support and work–family conflict: A meta-analysis clarifying the influence of general and work–family-specific supervisor and organizational support. *Personnel Psychology, 64*, 289–313. https://doi.org/10.1111/j.1744-6570.2011.01211.x

Kotter, J. P. (1995, March-April). Leading change: Why transformation efforts fail? *Harvard Business Review*, 59–67.

Kreiner, G. E., Hollensbe, E. C., & Sheep, M. L. (2009). Balancing borders and bridges: Negotiating the workhome interface via boundary work tactics. *Academy of Management Journal, 52*, 704–730. https://doi.org/10.5465/amj.2009.43669916

Kristof-Brown, A. L., Zimmerman, R. D., & Johnson, E. C. (2005). Consequences of individuals' fit at work: A meta-analysis of person-job, person-organization, person-group, and person-supervisor fit. *Personnel Psychology, 58*, 281–320. https://doi.org/10.1111/j.1744-6570.2005.00672.x

Kuijpers, E., Kooij, D. T., & van Woerkom, M. (2020). Align your job with yourself: The relationship between a job crafting intervention and work engagement, and the role of workload. *Journal of Occupational Health Psychology, 25*, 1–16. https://doi.org/10.1037/ocp0000175

Latack, J. C. (1986). Coping with job stress: Measures and future directions for scale development. *Journal of Applied Psychology, 71*, 377–385. https://doi.org/10.1037/0021-9010.71.3.377

Lazarus, R. S., & Folkman, S. (1987). Transactional theory and research on emotions and coping. *European Journal of Personality, 1*, 141–169. https://doi.org/10.1002/per.2410010304

Lewin, K., Lippitt, R., & White, R. (1939). Patterns of aggressive behavior in experimentally created "social climates". *Journal of Social Psychology, 10*, 269–299. https://doi.org/10.1080/00224545.1939.9713366

Li, Y., Chen, P. Y., Chen, F. L., & Chen, Y. L. (2017). Preventing school bullying: Investigation of the links between anti-bullying strategies, psychological ownership, prevention climate, and prevention leadership. *Applied Psychology, 66*, 577–598. https://doi.org/10.1111/apps.12107

Li, Y., Chen, P. Y., Tuckey, M. R., McLinton, S. S., & Dollard, M. F. (2019). Prevention through job design: Identifying high-risk job characteristics associated with workplace bullying. *Journal of Occupational Health Psychology, 24*, 297–306. https://doi.org/10.1037/ocp0000133

Liang, L. H., Coulombe, C., Brown, D. J., Lian, H., Hanig, S., Ferris, L., & Keeping, K. M. (2022). Can two wrongs make a right? The buffering effect of retaliation on subordinate well-being following abusive supervision. *Journal of Occupational Health Psychology, 27*(1), 37–52. https://doi.org/10.1037/ocp0000291

Lichtenthaler, P. W., &Fischbach, A. (2019). A meta-analysis on promotion- and prevention-focused job crafting. *European Journal of Work & Organizational Psychology, 28*, 30–50. https://doi.org/10.1080/1359432X.2018.1527767

Liu, C., Spector, P. E., & Shi, L. (2007). Cross-national job stress: A quantitative and qualitative study. *Journal of Organizational Behavior, 28*, 209–239. https://doi.org/10.1002/job.435

Locke, E. A., & Latham, G. P. (2002). Building a practically useful theory of goal setting and task motivation: A 35-year odyssey. *American Psychologist, 57*, 705–717. https://doi.org/10.1037/0003-066X.57.9.705

Logan, M. S., & Ganster, D. C. (2005). An experimental evaluation of a control intervention to alleviate job-related stress. *Journal of Management, 31*, 90–107. https://doi.org/10.1177/0149206304271383

Luchman, J. N., & González-Morales, M. G. (2013). Demands, control, and support: A meta-analytic review of work characteristics interrelationships. *Journal of Occupational Health Psychology, 18*, 37–52. https://doi.org/10.1037/a0030541

Marchand, A., Haines, V. Y., & Dextras-Gauthier, J. (2013). Quantitative analysis of organizational culture in occupational health research: A theory-based validation in 30 workplaces of the organizational culture profile instrument. *BMC Public Health, 13*, 443. https://doi.org/10.1186/1471-2458-13-443

Maslach, C., Schaufeli, W. B., & Leiter, M. P. (2001). Job burnout. *Annual Review of Psychology, 52,* 397–422. https://doi.org/10.1146/annurev.psych.52.1.397

Mathieu, M., Eschleman, K. J., & Cheng, D. (2019). Meta-analytic and multiwave comparison of emotional support and instrumental support in the workplace. *Journal of Occupational Health Psychology, 24,* 387–409. https://doi.org/10.1037/ocp0000135

Mayes, B. T., & Allen, R. W. (1977). Toward a definition of organizational politics. *Academy of Management Review, 2,* 672–678. https://doi.org/10.5465/amr.1977.4406753

McGrath, J. E. (1976). Stress and behavior in organizations. In M. D. Dunnette (Ed.), *Handbook of industrial and organizational psychology* (pp. 1351–1395). Rand McNally.

Michel, J. S., Kotrba, L. M., Mitchelson, J. K., Clark, M. A., & Baltes, B. B. (2011). Antecedents of work–family conflict: A meta-analytic review. *Journal of Organizational Behavior, 32,* 689–725. https://doi.org/10.1002/job.695

Michel, J. S., Mitchelson, J. K., Pichler, S., & Cullen, K. L. (2010). Clarifying relationships among work and family social support, stressors, and work–family conflict. *Journal of Vocational Behavior, 76,* 91–104. https://doi.org/10.1016/j.jvb.2009.05.007

Montano, D., Reeske, A., Franke, F., & Hüffmeier, J. (2017). Leadership, followers' mental health and job performance in organizations: A comprehensive meta-analysis from an occupational health perspective. *Journal of Organizational Behavior, 38,* 327–350. https://doi.org/10.1002/job.2124

Morgeson, F. P., & Humphrey, S. E. (2006). The Work Design Questionnaire (WDQ): Developing and validating a comprehensive measure for assessing job design and the nature of work. *Journal of Applied Psychology, 91,* 1321–1339. https://doi.org/10.1037/0021-9010.91.6.1321

Morral, A. R., Matthews, M., Cefalu, M., Schell, T. L., & Cottrell, L. (2021). *Effects of sexual assault and sexual harassment on separation from the U.S. military: Findings from the 2014 RAND Military Workplace Study.* RAND Corporation. https://apps.dtic.mil/sti/pdfs/AD1122542.pdf

Nahrgang, J. D., Morgeson, F. P., & Hofmann, D. A. (2011). Safety at work: A meta-analytic investigation of the link between job demands, job resources, burnout, engagement, and safety outcomes. *Journal of Applied Psychology, 96,* 71–94. https://doi.org/10.1037/a0021484

Nielsen, K., Randall, R., Holten, A., & González, E. R. (2010). Conducting organizational-level occupational health interventions: What works? *Work & Stress, 24,* 234–259. https://doi.org/10.1080/02678373.2010.515393

Nielsen, M. B., & Einarsen, S. (2012). Outcomes of exposure to workplace bullying: A meta-analytic review. *Work & Stress, 26,* 309–332. https://doi.org/10.1080/02678373.2012.734709

Nixon, A. E., Mazzola, J. J., Bauer, J., Krueger, J. R., & Spector, P. E. (2011). Can work make you sick? A meta-analysis of the relationships between job stressors and physical symptoms. *Work & Stress, 25,* 1–22. https://doi.org/10.1080/02678373.2011.569175

Noe, R. A., & Colquitt, J. A. (2002). Planning for training impact: Principles of training effectiveness. In K. Kraiger (Ed.), *Creating, implementing, and managing effective training and development* (pp. 53–79). Jossey-Bass.

Occupational Information Network. (2021). *Mental health counselors.* https://www.onetonline.org/link/summary/21-1014.00

Odle-Dusseau, H. N., Hammer, L. B., Crain, T. L., & Bodner, T. E. (2016). The influence of family-supportive supervisor training on employee job performance and attitudes: An organizational work–family intervention. *Journal of Occupational Health Psychology, 21,* 296–308. https://doi.org/10.1037/a0039961

Oprea, B. T., Barzin, L., Vîrgă, D., Iliescu, D., & Rusu, A. (2019). Effectiveness of job crafting interventions: A meta-analysis and utility analysis. *European Journal of Work and Organizational Psychology, 28,* 723–741. https://doi.org/10.1080/1359432X.2019.1646728

Örtqvist, D., & Wincent, J. (2006). Prominent consequences of role stress: A meta-analytic review. *International Journal of Stress Management, 13,* 399–422. https://doi.org/10.1037/1072-5245.13.4.399

Park, H. I., Jacob, A. C., Wagner, S. H., & Baiden, M. (2014). Job control and burnout: A meta-analytic test of the Conservation of Resources model. *Applied Psychology: An International Review, 63,* 607–642. https://doi.org/10.1111/apps.12008

Parker, S. K., Morgeson, F. P., & Johns, G. (2017). One hundred years of work design research: Looking back and looking forward. *Journal of Applied Psychology, 102,* 403–420. https://doi.org/10.1037/apl0000106

Parks, K. M., & Steelman, L. A. (2008). Organizational wellness programs: A meta-analysis. *Journal of Occupational Health Psychology, 13,* 58–68. https://doi.org/10.1037/1076-8998.13.1.58

Payne, R. L., Jabri, M. M., & Pearson, A. W. (1988). On the importance of knowing the affective meaning of job demands. *Journal of Organizational Behavior, 9,* 149–158. https://doi.org/10.1002/job.4030090206

Peters, L. H., & O'Connor, E. J. (1980). Situational constraints and work outcomes: The influences of a frequently overlooked construct. *Academy of Management Review, 5,* 391–397. https://doi.org/10.5465/amr.1980.4288856

Peters, L. H., O'Connor, E. J., & Rudolf, C. J. (1980). The behavioral and affective consequences of performance-relevant situational variables. *Organizational Behavior and Human Performance, 25,* 79–96. https://doi.org/10.1016/0030-5073(80)90026-4

Pfeffer, J., Vilendrer, S., Joseph, G., Kim, J., & Singer, S. J. (2020). Employers' role in employee health: Why they do what they do. *Journal of Occupational and Environmental Medicine, 62,* e601–e610. https://doi.org/10.1097/JOM.0000000000001967

Pindek, S., Demircioğlu, E., Howard, D. J., Eatough, E. M., & Spector, P. E. (2019). Illegitimate tasks are not created equal: Examining the effects of attributions on unreasonable and unnecessary tasks. *Work & Stress, 33,* 231–246. https://doi.org/10.1080/02678373.2018.1496160

Pindek, S. & Spector, P. E. (2016). Organizational constraints: A meta-analysis of a major stressor. *Work & Stress, 30,* 7–25. https://doi.org/10.1080/02678373.2015.1137376

Rafaeli, A., Erez, A., Ravid, S., Derfler-Rozin, R., Treister, D. E., & Scheyer, R. (2012). When customers exhibit verbal aggression, employees pay cognitive costs. *Journal of Applied Psychology, 97,* 931–950. https://doi.org/10.1037/a0028559

Richardson, K. M., & Rothstein, H. R. (2008). Effects of occupational stress management intervention programs: A meta-analysis. *Journal of Occupational Health Psychology, 13,* 69–93. https://doi.org/10.1037/1076-8998.13.1.69

Rudolph, C. W., Katz, I. M., Lavigne, K. N., & Zacher, H. (2017). Job crafting: A meta-analysis of relationships with individual differences, job characteristics, and work outcomes. *Journal of Vocational Behavior, 102,* 112–138. https://doi.org/10.1016/j.jvb.2017.05.008

Sauter, S. L., Murphy, L. R., & Hurrell, J. J. (1990). Prevention of work-related psychological disorders: A national strategy proposed by the National Institute for Occupational Safety and Health (NIOSH). *American Psychologist, 45,* 1146–1158. https://doi.org/10.1037/10108-002

Schall, M. C., & Chen, P. Y. (2021). Evidence-based strategies for improving occupational safety and health among teleworkers during and after the coronavirus pandemic. *Human Factors.* Advance online publication. https://doi.org/10.1177/0018720820984583

Schaufeli, W. B., Salanova, M., González-Romá, V., & Bakker, A. B. (2002). The measurement of engagement and burnout: A two sample confirmatory factor analytic approach. *Journal of Happiness Studies, 3,* 71–92. https://doi.org/10.1023/A:1015630930326

Schmidt, S., Roesler, U., Kusserow, T., & Rau, R. (2014). Uncertainty in the workplace: examining role ambiguity and role conflict, and their link to depression: A meta-analysis. *European Journal of Work and Organizational Psychology, 23*, 91–106. https://doi.org/10.1080/1359432X.2012.711523

Schmidt, B., Schneider, M., Seeger, P., van Vianen, A., Loerbroks, A., & Herr, R. M. (2019). A comparison of job stress models: Associations with employee well-being, absenteeism, presenteeism, and resulting costs. *Journal of Occupational and Environmental Medicine, 61*, 535–544. https://doi.org/10.1097/JOM.0000000000001582

Semmer, N. K., Jacobshagen, N., Meier, L. L., Elfering, A., Beehr, T. A., Kälin, W., & Tschan, F. (2015). Illegitimate tasks as a source of work stress. *Work and Stress, 29*, 32–56. https://doi.org/10.1080/02678373.2014.1003996

Siegrist, J. (1996). Adverse health effects of high-effort/low-reward conditions. *Journal of Occupational Health Psychology, 1*, 27–41. https://doi.org/10.1037/1076-8998.1.1.27

Smallwood, S. (2007). *Poetry performance on the occasion of Workers' Memorial Day 2007.* https://www.cdc.gov/niosh/docs/video/osh_poem.html

Sonnentag, S., & Frese, M. (2003). Stress in organizations. In W. C. Borman, D. R. Ilgen, & R. J. Klimonski (Eds.), *Handbook of psychology: Industrial and organizational psychology* (Vol. 12, pp. 453–491). John Wiley & Sons, Inc. https://doi.org/10.1002/0471264385.wei1218

Sonnentag, S., & Fritz, C. (2007). The recovery experience questionnaire: Development and validation of a measure for assessing recuperation and unwinding from work. *Journal of Occupational Health Psychology, 12*, 204–221. https://doi.org/10.1037/1076-8998.12.3.204

Sonnentag, S., & Fritz, C. (2015). Recovery from job stress: The stressor-detachment model as an integrative framework. *Journal of Organizational Behavior, 36*, S72–S103. https://doi.org/10.1002/job.1924

Sonnentag, S., & Lischetzke, T. (2018). Illegitimate tasks reach into afterwork hours: A multilevel study. *Journal of Occupational Health Psychology, 23*, 248–261. https://doi.org/10.1037/ocp0000077

Southern Poverty Law Center. (2016). *SPLC files federal safety complaints against poultry plant that fired whistleblowers.* https://www.splcenter.org/news/2016/07/26/splc-files-federal-safety-complaints-against-poultry-plant-fired-whistleblowers

Spector, P. E. (1986). Perceived control by employees: A meta-analysis of studies concerning autonomy and participation at work. *Human relations, 39*, 1005–1016. https://doi.org/10.1177/001872678603901104

Spector, P. E. (1998). A control theory of the job stress process. In C. L. Cooper (Ed.), *Theories of organizational stress* (pp. 153–169). Oxford University Press.

Spector, P. E. (2021, May 5). *How to build a healthier work organization.* https://paulspector.com/how-to-build-a-healthier-work-organization/

Spector, P. E., Jex, S. M., & Chen, P. Y. (1995). Relations of incumbent affect-related personality traits with incumbent and objective measures of characteristics of jobs. *Journal of Organizational Behavior, 16*, 59–65. https://doi.org/10.1002/job.4030160108

Spector, P. E., Zapf, D., Chen, P. Y., & Frese, M. (2000). Why negative affectivity should not be controlled in job stress research: Don't throw out the baby with the bath water. *Journal of Organizational Behavior, 21*, 79–95. https://www.jstor.org/stable/3100407 https://doi.org/10.1002/(SICI)1099-1379(200002)21:1<79::AID-JOB964>3.0.CO;2-G

Steed, L. B., Swider, B. W., Keem, S., & Liu, J. T. (2021). Leaving work at work: A meta-analysis on employee recovery from work. *Journal of Management, 47*, 867–897. https://doi.org/10.1177/0149206319864153

Stone, A. A., Neale, J. M., Cox, D. S., Napoli, A., Valdimarsdottir, H., & Kennedy-Moore, E. (1994). Daily events are associated with a secretory immune response to an oral antigen in men. *Health Psychology, 13*, 440–446. https://doi.org/10.1037/0278-6133.13.5.440

Stryker, S., & Burke, P. J. (2000). The past, present, and future of an identity theory. *Social Psychology Quarterly, 63*, 284–297. https://doi.org/10.2307/2695840

Tepper, B. J., & Zhou, Z. (2017). Abusive supervision. In S. G. Rogelbert (Ed.), *Encyclopedia of industrial/organizational psychology* (2nd ed.). Sage. https://doi.org/10.1146/annurev-orgpsych-041015-062539

Tubre, T. C., & Collins, J. M. (2000). Jackson and Schuler (1985) revisited: A meta-analysis of the relationships between role ambiguity, role conflict, and job performance. *Journal of Management, 26,* 155–169. https://doi.org/10.1177/014920630002600104

Tuckey, M. R., Li, Y. Chen, P. Y., Dollard, M. F., McLinton, S., Rogers, A., & Neall, A. M. (2015). *Prevention of workplace bullying through risk assessment: Final project report.* Asia Pacific Centre for Work Health and Safety. http://apo.org.au/node/64434

Tuckey, M. R., Li, Y., Neall, A. M., Chen, P. Y., Dollard, M. F., McLinton, S. S., Rogers, A., & Mattiske, J. (2022). Workplace bullying as an organizational problem: Spotlight on people management practices. *Journal of Occupational Health Psychology, 27,* 544–565. https://doi.org/10.1037/ocp0000335

US Bureau of Labor Statistics. (2021). *Labor force statistics from the Current Population Survey.* https://www.bls.gov/cps/tables.htm

US Equal Employment Opportunity Commission. (2016, June). Select task force on the study of harassment in the workplace. https://www.eeoc.gov/select-task-force-study-harassment-workplace#_Toc453686311

US Equal Employment Opportunity Commission. (2021, April). *Imperial Pacific pays $105,000 to settle EEOC sex discrimination, harassment and retaliation suit.* https://www.eeoc.gov/newsroom/imperial-pacific-pays-105000-settle-eeoc-sex-discrimination-harassment-and-retaliation

US Equal Employment Opportunity Commission (EEOC) v. New Breed Logistics. (2015). *No. 13–6250, 2015 U.S. App. LEXIS 6650* (6th Cir. Apr. 22, 2015).

US National Institute for Occupational Safety and Health. (2022). Promising practices for Total Worker Health. https://www.cdc.gov/niosh/twh/practices.html

Vanhove, A., Herian, M., Perez, A., Harms, P., & Lester, P. (2016). Can resilience be developed at work? A meta-analytic review of resilience-building programme effectiveness. *Journal of Occupational and Organizational Psychology, 89,* 278–307. https://doi.org/10.1111/joop.12123

van der Doef, M., & Maes, S. (1999). The job demand-control (-support) model and psychological well-being: A review of 20 years of empirical research. *Work & Stress, 13,* 87–114. https://doi.org/10.1080/026783799296084

van Vegchel, N., de Jonge, J., Bosma, H., & Schaufeli, W. (2005). Reviewing the effort-reward imbalance model: Drawing up the balance of 45 empirical studies. *Social Science & Medicine, 60,* 1117–1131. https://doi.org/10.1016/j.socscimed.2004.06.043

van Vianen, A. E. M. (2018). Person–environment fit: A review of its basic tenets. *Annual Review of Organizational Psychology and Organizational Behavior, 5,* 75–101. https://doi.org/10.1146/annurev-orgpsych-032117-104702

Verbeek, J., Ruotsalainen, J., Laitinen, J., Korkiakangas, E., Lusa, S., Mänttäri, S., & Oksanen, T. (2019). Interventions to enhance recovery in healthy workers: A scoping review. *Occupational Medicine, 69,* 54–63. https://doi.org/10.1093/occmed/kqy141

Villanova, P., & Roman, M. A. (1993). A meta-analytic review of situational constraints and work-related outcomes: Alternative approaches to conceptualization. *Human Resource Management Review, 3,* 147–175. https://doi.org/10.1016/1053-4822(93)90021-U

Viswesvaran, C., Sanchez, J. I., & Fisher, J. (1999). The role of social support in the process of work stress: A meta-analysis. *Journal of Vocational Behavior, 54,* 314–334. https://doi.org/10.1006/jvbe.1998.1661

Webster, J. R., Beehr, T. A., & Love, K. (2011). Extending the challenge-hindrance model of occupational stress: The role of appraisal. *Journal of Vocational Behavior, 79,* 505–516. https://doi.org/10.1016/j.jvb.2011.02.001

Wiegand, D. M., Chen, P. Y., Hurrell, J. J., Jr., Jex, S., Nakata, A., Nigam, J. A., Robertson, M., & Tetrick, L. E. (2012). A consensus method for updating psychosocial measures used in NIOSH health hazard evaluations. *Journal of Occupational and Environmental Medicine, 54,* 350–355. https://doi.org/10.1097/JOM.0b013e3182440a04

World Health Organization. (2019). *International statistical classification of diseases and related health problems – 11th revision (ICD-*11). https://www.who.int/classifications/icd/en/

Wrzesniewski, A., & Dutton, J. E. (2001). Crafting a Job: Revisioning employees as active crafters of their work. *Academy of Management Review, 26,* 179–201. https://doi.org/10.5465/amr.2001.4378011

Yang, L. Q., Caughlin, D. E., Gazica, M. W., Truxillo, D. M., & Spector, P. E. (2014). Workplace mistreatment climate and potential employee and organizational outcomes: A meta-analytic review from the target's perspective. *Journal of Occupational Health Psychology, 19,* 315–335. https://doi.org/10.1037/a0036905

Zimmerman, F. H. (2012). Cardiovascular disease and risk factors in law enforcement personnel: A comprehensive review. *Cardiology in Review, 20,* 159–166. https://doi.org/10.1097/CRD.0b013e318248d631

# 8

# Appendix: Tools and Resources

**The following materials for your book can be downloaded free of charge once you register on the Hogrefe website:**

The following resources are for providers who want to learn more about chronic illness and caregiving. All clinicians are highly encouraged to be familiar with the links offered in Appendix 1 before they are offered to any client. No endorsement is intended or made of any external link, product, service, or information either by its inclusion or exclusion from this page or site. All critical information should be independently verified.

Appendix 1: Self-Report Outcome Measures
Appendix 2: Self-Report Resource Measures
Appendix 3: Self-Report Job Stressor Measures

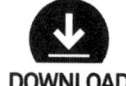

**DOWNLOAD**

**How to proceed:**

1. Go to www.hgf.io/media and create a user account. If you already have one, please log in.

2. Go to **My supplementary materials** in your account dashboard and enter the code below. You will automatically be redirected to the download area, where you can access and download the supplementary materials.

**Code: B-KUQF8C**

To make sure you have permanent direct access to all the materials, we recommend that you download them and save them on your computer.

# Appendix 1: Self-Report Outcome Measures

## Physical Self-Report Outcome Measures

### Physical and Mental Health

Frone, M. R. (2007). Obesity and absenteeism among U.S. workers: Do physical health and mental health explain the relation? *Journal of Workplace Behavioral Health, 22,* 65–79. https://doi.org/10.1080/15555240802157403

Veit, C. T., & Ware, J. E., Jr. (1983). The structure of psychological distress and well-being in general populations. *Journal of Counseling and Clinical Psychology, 51,* 730–742. https://doi.org/10.1037/0022-006X.51.5.730

Banks, M. H., Clegg, C. W., Jackson, P. R., Kemp, N. J., Stafford, E. M., & Wall, T. D. (1980). The use of the General Health Questionnaire as an indicator of mental health in occupational studies. *Journal of Occupational Psychology, 53,* 187–194. https://doi.org/10.1111/j.2044-8325.1980.tb00024.x

### Physical Symptoms

Schat, A. C., Kelloway, E. K., & Desmarais, S. (2005). The Physical Health Questionnaire (PHQ): Construct validation of a self-report scale of somatic symptoms. *Journal of Occupational Health Psychology, 10,* 363–381. https://doi.org/10.1037/1076-8998.10.4.363

Spector, P. E., & Jex, S. M. (1998). Development of four self-report measures of job stressors and strain: Interpersonal conflict at work scale, organizational constraints scale, quantitative workload inventory, and physical symptoms inventory. *Journal of Occupational Health Psychology, 3,* 356–367. https://doi.org/10.1037//1076-8998.3.4.356

### Sleep (Quantity, Quality, Inconsistency)

Flo, E., Bjorvatn, B., Folkard, S., Moen, B. E., Grønli, J., Nordhus, I. H., & Pallesen, S. (2012). A reliability and validity study of the Bergen Shift Work Sleep Questionnaire in nurses working three-shift rotations. *Chronobiology International, 29,* 937–946. https://doi.org/10.3109/07420528.2012.699120

Hoddes, E., Zarcone, V., Smythe, H., Phillips, R., & Dement, W. C. (1973). Quantification of sleepiness: A new approach. *Psychophysiology, 10,* 431–436. https://doi.org/10.1111/j.1469-8986.1973.tb00801.x

Jenkins, C. D., Stanton, B.-A., Niemcryk, S. J., & Rose, R. M. (1988). A scale for the estimation of sleep problems in clinical research. *Journal of Clinical Epidemiology, 41,* 313–321. https://doi.org/10.1016/0895-4356(88)90138-2

Johns, M. W. (1991). A new method for measuring daytime sleepiness: The Epworth Sleepiness Scale. *Sleep, 14,* 540–545. https://doi.org/10.1093/sleep/14.6.540

Mastin, D. F., Bryson, J., & Corwyn, R. (2006). Assessment of sleep hygiene using the Sleep Hygiene Index. *Journal of Behavioral Medicine, 29,* 223–227. https://doi.org/10.1007/s10865-006-9047-6

## Psychological Self-Report Outcome Measures

### Affect or Mood

Scollon, C., Diener, E., Oishi, S., & Biswas-Diener, R. (2005). An experience sampling and cross-cultural investigation of the relation between pleasant and unpleasant affect. *Cognition & Emotion, 19,* 27–52. https://doi.org/10.1080/02699930441000076

Watson, D., Clark. L. A., & Tellegen, A. (1988). Development and validation of brief measures of positive and negative affect: The PANAS scales. *Journal of Personality & Social Psychology, 54,* 1063–1070. https://doi.org/doi: 10.1037//0022-3514.54.6.1063

### Burnout and Engagement

Barrick, M. R., Thurgood, G. R., Smith, T. A., & Courtright, S. H. (2015). Collective organizational engagement: Linking motivational antecedents, strategic implementation, and firm performance. *Academy of Management Journal, 58,* 111–135. https://doi.org/10.5465/amj.2013.0227

Maslach, C., & Leiter, M. P. (2008). Early predictors of job burnout and engagement. *Journal of Applied Psychology, 93,* 498–512. https://doi.org/10.1037/0021-9010.93.3.498

Schaufeli, W., & Bakker, A. (2004). Utrecht Work Engagement Scale (UWES). https://www.wilmarschaufeli.nl/publications/Schaufeli/Test%20Manuals/Test_manual_UWES_English.pdf

Shirom, A., & Melamed, S. (2006). A comparison of the construct validity of two burnout measures in two groups of professionals. *International Journal of Stress Management, 13,* 176–200. https://doi.org/10.1037/1072-5245.13.2.176

### Boredom

Melamed, S., Ben-Avi, I., Luz, J., Green, M. S. (1995). Objective and subjective work monotony: Effects on job satisfaction, psychological distress, and absenteeism in blue-collar workers. *Journal of Applied Psychology, 80,* 29–42. https://doi.org/10.1037/0021-9010.80.1.29

See p. 78 for instructions on how to obtain the full-sized, printable PDF.

### Commitment

Allen, N. J., & Meyer, J. P. (1996). Affective, continuance, and normative commitment to the organization: An examination of construct validity. *Journal of Vocational Behavior, 49*, 252-276. https://doi.org/10.1006/jvbe.1996.0043

Mowday, R. T., Steers, R. M., & Porter, L. W. (1979). The measurement of organizational commitment. *Journal of Vocational Behavior, 14*, 224-247. https://doi.org/10.1016/0001-8791(79)90072-1

### Detachment From Work

Sonnentag, S., & Fritz, C. (2007). The Recovery Experience Questionnaire: Development and validation of a measure for assessing recuperation and unwinding from work. *Journal of Occupational Health Psychology, 12*, 204 – 221. https://doi.org/10.1037/1076-8998.12.3.204

### Engagement

Schaufeli, W. B., Salanova, M., González-Romá, V., & Bakker, A. B. (2002). The measurement of engagement and burnout: A two sample confirmatory factor analytic approach. *Journal of Happiness Studies, 3*, 71-92. https://doi.org/10.1023/A:1015630930326

### Fatigue

Frone, M. R., & Tidwell, M., -C., O. (2015). The meaning and measurement of work fatigue: Development and evaluation of the three-dimensional work fatigue inventory (3D-WFI). *Journal of Occupational Health Psychology, 20*, 273-288. https://doi.org/10.1037/a0038700

### Frustration

Peters, L. H., O'Connor, E. J., & Rudolf, C. J. (1980). The behavioral and affective consequences of performance-relevant situational variables. *Organizational Behavior and Human Performance, 25*, 79-96. https://doi.org/10.1016/0030-5073(80)90026-4

### Job Involvement

Kanungo, R. N. (1982). Measurement of job and work involvement. *Journal of Applied Psychology, 67*, 341-349. https://doi.org/10.1037/0021-9010.67.3.341

### Job Satisfaction

Bowling, N. A., & Hammond, G. D. (2008). A meta-analytic examination of the construct validity of the Michigan Organizational Assessment Questionnaire Job Satisfaction Subscale. *Journal of Vocational Behavior, 73*, 63-77. https://doi.org/10.1016/j.jvb.2008.01.004

Gregson, T. (1990). Measuring job satisfaction with a multiple-choice format of the job descriptives index. *Psychological Reports, 66*, 77-79. https://doi.org/10.2466/pr0.1990.66.3.787

Smith, P. C., Kendall, L., & Hulin, C. L. (1969). *The measurement of satisfaction in work and retirement.* Rand McNally.

Spector, P. E. (2022). *Job satisfaction: From assessment to intervention.* Routledge. https://doi.org/10.4324/9781003250616

### Life Satisfaction

Diener, E., Emmons, R. A., & Larsen, R. J. (1985). The satisfaction with life scale. *Journal of Personality Assessment, 49*, 71-75. https://doi.org/10.1207/s15327752jpa4901_13

### Organizational Depression

Bianchi, R., & Schonfeld, I. S. (2020). The Occupational Depression Inventory: A new tool for clinicians and epidemiologists. *Journal of Psychosomatic Research, 138*, 110249. https://doi.org/10.1016/j.jpsychores.2020.110249

### Perceived Stress

Chen, P. Y., & Spector, P. E. (1991). Negative affectivity as the underlying cause of correlations between stressors and strains. *Journal of Applied Psychology, 76*, 398-407. https://doi.org/10.1037/0021-9010.76.3.398

Kamarck, T., & Mermelstein, R. (1983). A global measure of perceived stress. *Journal of Health and Social Behavior, 24*, 385-396. https://doi.org/10.2307/2136404

### Rumination

Frone, M. R. (2015). Relations of negative and positive work experiences to employee alcohol use: Testing the intervening role of negative and positive work rumination. *Journal of Occupational Health Psychology, 20*, 148-160. https://doi.org/10.1037/a0038375

Mohr, G., Müller, A., Rigotti, T., Aycan, Z., & Tschan, F. (2006). The assessment of psychological strain in work contexts. *European Journal of Psychological Assessment, 22*, 198-206. https://doi.org/10.1027/1015-5759.22.3.198

See p. 78 for instructions on how to obtain the full-sized, printable PDF.

### State Anger and Anxiety

Chen, P. Y., & Spector, P. E. (1991). Negative affectivity as the underlying cause of correlations between stressors and strains. *Journal of Applied Psychology, 76*, 398–407. https://doi.org/10.1037/0021-9010.76.3.398

Spector, P. E., Dwyer, D. J., & Jex, S. M. (1988). Relation of job stressors to affective, health, and performance outcomes: A comparison of multiple data sources. *Journal of Applied Psychology, 73*, 11–19. https://doi.org/10.1037/0021-9010.73.1.11

### Well-Being

Van Katwyk, P. T., Fox, S., Spector, P. E., & Kelloway, E. K. (2000). Using the Job-Related Affective Well-Being Scale (JAWS) to investigate affective responses to work stressors. *Journal of Occupational Health Psychology, 5*, 219–230. https://doi.org/10.1037/1076-8998.5.2.219

## Behavioral Self-Report Outcome Measures

### Counterproductive, Deviant, Antisocial, or Aggressive Behaviors

Bennett, R. J., & Robinson, S. L. (2000). Development of a measure of workplace deviance. *Journal of Applied Psychology, 85*, 349–360. https://doi.org/10.1037/0021-9010.85.3.349

Robinson, S. L., & O'Leary-Kelly, A. M. (1998). Monkey see, monkey do: The influence of work groups on the antisocial behavior of employees. *Academy of Management Journal, 41*, 658–672. https://doi.org/10.5465/256963

Spector, P. E., Fox, S., Penney, L. M., Bruursema, K., Goh, A., & Kessler, S. (2006). The dimensionality of counterproductivity: Are all counterproductive behaviors created equal? *Journal of Vocational Behavior, 68*, 446–460. https://doi.org/10.1016/j.jvb.2005.10.005

### Health Behaviors (Smoking, Caffeinated Beverage/Alcohol/High Fat or Sugar Snack Consumption, Food Intake, Exercises)

Caan, B., Coates, A., & Schaffer, D. (1995). Variations in sensitivity, specificity, and predictive value of a dietary fat screener modified from Block et al. *Journal of the American Dietetic Association, 95*, 564–568. https://doi.org/10.1016/S0002-8223(95)00153-0

Craig, C. L., Marshall, A. L., Sjostrom, M., Bauman, A. E., Booth, M. L., Ainsworth, B. E., Pratt, M., Ekelund, U., Yngve, A., Sallis, J. F., & Oja, P. (2003). International Physical Activity Questionnaire: 12-country reliability and validity. *Medicine and Science in Sports and Exercise, 35*, 1381–1395. https://doi.org/10.1249/01.MSS.0000078924.61453.FB

Frone, M. R., Russell, M., & Cooper, M. L. (1993). Relationship of work-family conflict, gender, and alcohol expectancies to alcohol use/abuse. *Journal of Organizational Behavior, 14*, 545–558. https://doi.org/10.1002/job.4030140604

Grzywacz, J. G., & Marks, N. F. (2001). Social inequalities and exercise during adulthood: Toward an ecological perspective. *Journal of Health and Social Behavior, 42*, 202–220. https://doi.org/10.2307/3090178

Jones, F., O'Connor, D. B., Conner, M., McMillan, B., & Ferguson, E. (2007). Impact of daily mood, work hours, and iso-strain variables on self-reported health behaviors. *Journal of Applied Psychology, 92*, 1731–1740. https://doi.org/10.1037/0021-9010.92.6.1731

### Job Performance

Farh, J. L., Dobbins, G. H., & Cheng, B. S. (1991). Cultural relativity in action: A comparison of self-ratings made by Chinese and US workers. *Personnel Psychology, 44*, 129–147. https://doi.org/10.1111/j.1744-6570.1991.tb00693.x

Motowidlo, S. J., & Van Scotter, J. R. (1994). Evidence that task performance should be distinguished from contextual performance. *Journal of Applied Psychology, 79*, 475–480. https://doi.org/10.1037/0021-9010.79.4.475

### Presenteeism and Absenteeism

Koopman, C., Pelletier, K. R., Murray, J. F., Sharda, C. E., Berger, M. L., Turpin, R. S., Hackleman, P. Gibson, P., Holmes, D. M., & Bendel, T. (2002). Stanford presenteeism scale: health status and employee productivity. *Journal of Occupational and Environmental Medicine, 44*, 14–20. https://doi.org/10.1097/00043764-200201000-00004

### Proactive Work Behavior

Parker, S. K., & Collins, C. G. (2010). Taking stock: Integrating and differentiating multiple proactive behaviors. *Journal of Management, 36*, 633–662. https://doi.org/10.1177/0149206308321554

### Resilience

Friborg, O., Hjemdal, O., Rosenvinge, J. H., & Martinussen, M. (2003). A new rating scale for adult resilience: what are the central protective resources behind healthy adjustment? *International Journal of Methods in Psychiatric Research, 12*, 65–76. https://doi.org/10.1002/mpr.143

### Withdrawal (Absenteeism, Lateness)

Borofsky, G. L. (2000). Predicting involuntary dismissal for unauthorized absence, lateness, and poor performance in the selection of unskilled and semiskilled British contract factory operatives: The contribution of the Employee Reliability Inventory. *Psychological Reports, 87*, 95–104. https://doi.org/10.2466/pr0.2000.87.1.95

See p. 78 for instructions on how to obtain the full-sized, printable PDF.

Kessler, R. C., Barber, C., Beck, A., Berglund, P., Cleary, P. D., McKenas, D., Pronk, N., Simon, G., Stang, P., Ustun, T. B., & Wang, P. (2003). The World Health Organization Health and Work Performance Questionnaire (HPQ). *Journal of Occupational and Environmental Medicine, 45,* 156–174. https://doi.org/10.1097/01.jom.0000052967.43131.51

Hanisch, K. A., & Hulin, C. L. (1990). Job attitudes and organizational withdrawal: An examination of retirement and other voluntary withdrawal behaviors. *Journal of Vocational Behavior, 37,* 60–78. https://doi.org/10.1016/0001-8791(90)90007-O

Paget, K. J., Lang, D. L., & Shultz, K. S. (1998). Development and validation of an employee absenteeism scale. *Psychological Reports, 82,* 1144–1146. https://doi.org/10.2466/pr0.1998.82.3c.1144

### Turnover Intention

Wayne, S. J., Shore, L. M., & Linden, R. C. (1997). Perceived organizational support and leader member exchange: A social exchange perspective. *Academy of Management Journal, 40,* 82–111. https://doi.org/10.5465/257021

## Family Self-Report Outcome Measures

### Adolescent Problem Behaviors

Galambos, N. L., Sears, H. A., Almeida, D. M., & Kolaric, G. C. (1995). Parents' work overload and problem behavior in young adolescents. *Journal of Research on Adolescence, 5,* 201–223. https://doi.org/10.1207/s15327795jra0502_3

### Child Health and Physical Activity

Johnson, R. C., & Allen, T. D. (2013). Examining the links between employed mothers' work characteristics, physical activity, and child health. *Journal of Applied Psychology, 98,* 148–157. https://doi.org/10.1037/a0030460

### Family Performance

Frone, M. R., Yardley, J. K., & Markel, K. S. (1997). Developing and testing an integrative model of the work-family interface. *Journal of Vocational Behavior, 50,* 145–167. https://doi.org/10.1006/jvbe.1996.1577

### Family Satisfaction

Aryee, S., Luk, V, Leung, A., & Lo, S. (1999). Role stressors, interrole conflict, and well-being: The moderating influence of spousal support and coping behaviors among employed parents in Hong Kong. *Journal of Vocational Behavior, 54,* 259–278. https://doi.org/10.1006/jvbe.1998.1667

### Marital Adjustment

Beatty, C. A. (1996). The stress of managerial and professional women: Is the price too high? *Journal of Organizational Behavior, 17,* 233–251. https://doi.org/10.1002/(SICI)1099-1379(199605)17:3<233::AID-JOB746>3.0.CO;2-V

### Marital Stress

Guelzow, M. G., Bird, G. Q., & Koball, E. H. (1991). An exploratory path analysis of the stress process for dual-career men and women. *Journal of Marriage and the Family, 53,* 151–164. https://doi.org/10.2307/353140

### Marital Satisfaction

Netemeyer, R. G., Boles, J. S., & McMurrian, R. (1996). Development and validation of work-family conflicts and work-family conflict scales. *Journal of Applied Psychology, 81,* 400–410. https://doi.org/10.1037/0021-9010.81.4.400

### Quality of Family Life

Higgins, C. A., & Duxbury, L. E. (1992). Work-family conflict: A comparison of dual-career and traditional career men. *Journal of Organizational Behavior, 13,* 389–411. https://doi.org/10.1002/job.4030130407

### Parental Satisfaction

Kinnunen, U., & Mauno, S. (1998). Antecedents and outcomes of work-family conflict among employed women and men in Finland. *Human Relations, 51,* 157–177. https://doi.org/10.1177/001872679805100203

### Parenting Behaviors

Stewart, W., & Barling, J. (1996). Fathers' work experiences effect children's behaviors via job-related affect and parenting behaviors. *Journal of Organizational Behavior, 17,* 221–232. https://doi.org/10.1002/(SICI)1099-1379(199605)17:3<221::AID-JOB741>3.0.CO;2-G

### Satisfaction With Leisure Activities

Rice, R. W, Frone, M. R., & McFarlin, D. B. (1992). Work-nonwork conflict and the perceived quality of life. *Journal of Organizational Behavior, 13,* 155–168. https://doi.org/10.1002/job.4030130205

See p. 78 for instructions on how to obtain the full-sized, printable PDF.

# Appendix 2: Self-Report Resource Measures

### Assertiveness

Demerouti, E., Van Eeuwijk, E., Snelder, M., & Wild, U. (2011). Assessing the effects of a "personal effectiveness" training on psychological capital, assertiveness and self-awareness using self-other agreement. *The Career Development International, 16,* 60-81. https://doi.org/10.1108/13620431111107810

### Coping

Carver, C. S., Scheier, M. F., & Weintraub, J. K. (1989). Assessing coping strategies: a theoretically based approach. *Journal of Personality and Social Psychology, 56,* 267-283. https://doi.org/10.1037/0022-3514.56.2.267

Folkman, S., Lazarus, R. S., Dunkel-Schetter, C., DeLongis, A., & Gruen, R. J. (1986). Dynamics of a stressful encounter: Cognitive appraisal, coping, and encounter outcomes. *Journal of Personality and Social Psychology, 50,* 992-1003. https://doi.org/10.1037/0022-3514.50.5.992

Latack, J. C. (1986). Coping with job stress: Measures and future directions for scale development. *Journal of Applied Psychology, 71,* 377-385. https://doi.org/10.1037/0021-9010.71.3.377

Latack, J. C., & Havlovic, S. J. (1992). Coping with job stress: A conceptual evaluation framework for coping measures. *Journal of Organizational Behavior, 13,* 479-508. https://doi.org/10.1002/job.4030130505

### Job Crafting

Slemp, G. R., & Vella-Brodrick, D. A. (2013). The job crafting questionnaire: A new scale to measure the extent to which employees engage in job crafting. *International Journal of Wellbeing, 3,* 126-146. https://doi.org/10.5502/ijw.v3i2.1

Tims, M., Bakker, A. B., & Derks, D. (2012). Development and validation of the job crafting scale. *Journal of Vocational Behavior, 80,* 173-186. https://doi.org/10.1016/j.jvb.2011.05.009

### Family Supportive Supervisor Behaviors

Hammer, L. B., Kossek, E. E., Yragui, N. L., Bodner, T. E., & Hanson, G. C. (2009). Development and validation of a multidimensional measure of family supportive supervisor behaviors (FSSB). *Journal of Management, 35,* 837-856. https://doi.org/10.1177/0149206308328510

Hammer, L. B., Ernst Kossek, E., Bodner, T., & Crain, T. (2013). Measurement development and validation of the Family Supportive Supervisor Behavior Short-Form (FSSB-SF). *Journal of Occupational Health Psychology, 18,* 285-296. https://doi.org/10.1037/a0032612

### Motivational Task, Knowledge, Social, and Contextual Characteristics

Morgeson, F. P., & Humphrey, S. E. (2006). The Work Design Questionnaire (WDQ): Developing and validating a comprehensive measure for assessing job design and the nature of work. *Journal of Applied Psychology, 91,* 1321-1339. https://doi.org/10.1037/0021-9010.91.6.1321

### Optimism

Scheier, M. F., Carver, C. S., & Bridges, M. W. (2001). Optimism, pessimism, and psychological well-being. In E. C. Chang (Ed.), *Optimism and pessimism: Implications for theory, research, and practice* (pp. 189-216). American Psychological Association.

### Organizational, Supervisor, Coworker, Family-Friend Support

Beehr, T. A., King, L. A., & King, D. W. (1990). Social support and occupational stress: Talking to supervisors. *Journal of Vocational Behavior, 36,* 61-81. https://doi.org/10.1016/0001-8791(90)90015-T

Caplan, R. D., Cobb, S., French, J. R. P., Harrison, R. V., & Pinneau, S. R., Jr. (1975). *Job demands and worker health* (Publication No. 75-160). DHEW (NIOSH).

Eisenberger, R., Huntington, R., Hutchison, S., & Sowa, D. (1986). Perceived organizational support. *Journal of Applied Psychology, 71,* 500-507. https://doi.org/10.1037/0021-9010.71.3.500

### Recovery

Sonnentag, S., & Fritz, C. (2007). The recovery experience questionnaire: Development and validation of a measure for assessing recuperation and unwinding from work. *Journal of Occupational Health Psychology, 12,* 204-221. https://doi.org/10.1037/1076-8998.12.3.204

See p. 78 for instructions on how to obtain the full-sized, printable PDF.

### Resilience

Block, J., & Kremen, A. M. (1996). IQ and ego-resiliency: Conceptual and empirical connections and separateness. *Journal of Personality and Social Psychology, 70,* 349–361. https://doi.org/10.1037/0022-3514.70.2.349

### Self-Efficacy

Schwarzer, R., & Jerusalem, M. (1995). Generalized self-efficacy scale. In J. Weinman, S. Wright, & M. Johnston (Eds.), *Measures in health psychology: A user's portfolio. Causal and control beliefs* (pp. 35–37). Nfer-Nelson.

### Self-Esteem

Pierce, J. L., Gardner, D. G., Cummings, L. L., & Dunham, R. B. (1989). Organizational-based self-esteem: Construct definition, measurement, and validation. *Academy of Management Journal, 32,* 622–648. https://doi.org/10.5465/256437

### Work Locus of Control

Spector, P. E. (1988). Development of the work locus of control scale. *Journal of Occupational Psychology, 61,* 335–340. https://doi.org/10.1111/j.2044-8325.1988.tb00470.x

See p. 78 for instructions on how to obtain the full-sized, printable PDF.

# Appendix 3: Self-Report Job Stressor Measures

### Workplace Mistreatment

Nixon, A. E., Arvan, M., & Spector, P. E. (2021). Will the real mistreatment please stand up? Examining the assumptions and measurement of bullying and incivility. *Work & Stress, 35*, 398-422. https://doi.org/10.1080/02678373.2021.1891584

### Abusive Supervisor

Tepper, B. J., Henle, C. A., Lambert, L. S., Giacalone, R. A., & Duffy, M. K. (2008). Abusive supervision and subordinates' organization deviance. *Journal of Applied Psychology, 93*, 721-732. https://doi.org/10.1037/0021-9010.93.4.721

### Sexual Harassment and Gender Harassment

Fitzgerald, L. F., Gelfand, M. J., & Drasgow, F. (1995). Measuring sexual harassment: Theoretical and psychometric advances. *Basic and Applied Social Psychology, 17,* 425-427. https://doi.org/10.1207/s15324834basp1704_2

Fitzgerald, L. F., Shullman, S. L., Bailey, N., Richards, M., Swecker, J. Gold, A., Ormerod, A. J., & Weitzman, L. (1988). The incidence and dimensions of sexual harassment in academia and the workplace. *Journal of Vocational Behavior, 32,* 152-175. https://doi.org/10.1016/0001-8791(88)90012-7

### Workplace Bullying

Elo, A.-L., Dallner, M., Gamberale, F., Hottinen, V., Knardahl, S., Lindström, K., Skogstad, A., & Ørhede, E. (2000). Validation of the Nordic Questionnaire for Psychological and Social Factors at Work–QPSNordic. In M. Vartiainen, F. Avallone, & N. Anderson (Eds.), *Innovative theories, tools, and practices in work and organizational psychology* (pp. 47-57). Hogrefe & Huber Publishers.

Nielsen, M. B., Notelaers, G., & Einarsen, S. (2011). Measuring exposure to workplace bullying. In S. Einarsen, H. Hoel, D. Zapf, & C. L. Cooper (Eds), *Bullying and emotional abuse in the workplace. Developments in theory, research and practice* (pp. 149-174). CRC Press.

### Workplace Incivility

Cortina, L. M., Magley, V. J., Williams, J. H., & Langhout, R. D. (2001). Incivility in the workplace: Incidence and impact. *Journal of Occupational Health Psychology, 6,* 64-80. https://doi.org/10.1037/1076-8998.6.1.64

Lim, S., & Cortina, L. M. (2005). Interpersonal mistreatment in the workplace: The interface and impact of general incivility and sexual harassment. *Journal of Applied Psychology, 90,* 483-496. https://doi.org/10.1037/0021-9010.90.3.483

### Workplace Ostracism

Ferris, D. L., Brown, D. J., Berry, J., & Lian, H. (2008). The development and validation of the Workplace Ostracism Scale. *Journal of Applied Psychology, 93,* 1348-1366. https://doi.org/10.1037/a0012743

Hitlan, R. T., & Noel, J. (2009). The influence of workplace exclusion and personality on counterproductive work behaviours: An interactionist perspective. *European Journal of Work and Organizational Psychology, 18,* 477-502. https://doi.org/10.1080/13594320903025028

### Emotional Labor

Zapf, D., Vogt, C., Seifert, C., Mertini, H., & Isic, A. (1990). Emotion work as a source of stress. The concept and the development of an instrument. *European Journal of Work and Organizational Psychology, 8,* 371-400. https://doi.org/10.1080/135943299398230

### Illegitimate Tasks

Semmer, N. K., Tschan, F., Meier, L. L., Facchin, S., & Jacobshagen, N. (2010). Illegitimate tasks and counterproductive work behavior. *Applied Psychology: An International Review, 59,* 70-96. https://doi.org/10.1111/j.1464-0597.2009.00416.x

### Interpersonal Conflict

Spector, P. E., & Jex, S. M. (1998). Development of four self-report measures of job stressors and strain: Interpersonal Conflict at Work Scale, Organizational Constraints Scale, Quantitative Workload Inventory, and Physical Symptoms Inventory. *Journal of Occupational Health Psychology, 3,* 356-367. https://doi.org/10.1037//1076-8998.3.4.356

See p. 78 for instructions on how to obtain the full-sized, printable PDF.

### Job Autonomy or Job Control

Jackson, P. R., Wall, T. D., Martin, R., & Davids, K. (1993). New measures of job control, cognitive demand, and production responsibility. *Journal of Applied Psychology, 78,* 753–762. https://doi.org/10.1037/0021-9010.78.5.753

Ng, K.-Y., Ang, S., & Chan, K.-Y. (2008). Personality and leader effectiveness: A moderated mediation model of leadership self-efficacy, job demands and job autonomy. *Journal of Applied Psychology, 93,* 733–743. https://doi.org/10.1037/0021-9010.93.4.733

### Job Demands

Karasek, R. A. (1979). Job demands, job decision latitude and mental strain: Implications for job redesign. *Administrative Science Quarterly, 24,* 285–308. https://doi.org/10.2307/2392498

### Job Insecurity

Lee, C., Bobko, P., Ashford, S. J., Chen, Z. X., & Ren, X. P. (2008). Cross-cultural development of an abridged job insecurity measure. *Journal of Organizational Behavior, 29,* 373–390. https://doi.org/10.1002/job.513

### Organizational or Situational Constraints

Peters, L., & O'Connor, E. (1980). Situational constraints and work outcomes: The influences of a frequently overlooked construct. *Academy of Management Review, 5,* 391–397. https://doi.org/10.5465/amr.1980.4288856

Spector, P. E., & Jex, S. M. (1998). Developmental of four self-report measures of job stressors and strain: Interpersonal conflict at work scale, organizational constraints scale, quantitative workload inventory, and physical symptoms inventory. *Journal of Occupational Health Psychology, 3,* 356–367. https://doi.org/10.1037//1076-8998.3.4.356

### Organizational Injustices

Cropanzano, R., Prehar, C. A., & Chen, P. Y. (2002). Using social exchange theory to distinguish procedural from interactional justice. *Group and Organization Management: An International Journal, 27,* 324–351. https://doi.org/10.1177/1059601102027003002

### Organizational Politics

Kacmar, K. M., & Ferris, G. R. (1991). Perceptions of organizational politics scale (POPS): Development and construct validation. *Education and Psychological Measurement, 51,* 193–205. https://doi.org/10.1177/0013164491511019

Ferris, G. R., & Kacmar, K. M. (1992). Perceptions of organizational politics. *Journal of Management, 18,* 93–116. https://doi.org/10.1177/014920639201800107

### Person–Organizational Fit

Bretz, R. B., & Judge, T. A. (1994). Person-organization fit and the theory of work adjustment: Implications for satisfaction, tenure, and career success. *Journal of Vocational Behavior, 44,* 32–54. https://doi.org/10.1006/jvbe.1994.1003

### Role Conflict, Ambiguity, and Overload

Rizzo, J. R., House, R. J., & Lirtzman, S. I. (1970). Role conflict and ambiguity in complex organizations. *Administrative Science Quarterly, 15,* 150–163. https://doi.org/10.2307/2391486

### Telepressure

Barber, L. K., & Santuzzi, A. M. (2015). Please respond ASAP: Workplace telepressure and employee recovery. *Journal of Occupational Health Psychology, 20,* 172–189. https://doi.org/10.1037/a0038278

### Work–Family Conflict

Carlson, D. S., Kacmar, K. M., & Williams, L. J. (2000). Construction and initial validation of a multidimensional measure of work-family conflict. *Journal of Vocational Behavior, 56,* 249–276. https://doi.org/10.1006/jvbe.1999.1713

See p. 78 for instructions on how to obtain the full-sized, printable PDF.

Netemeyer, R. G., Boles, J. S., & McMurrian, R. (1996). Development and validation of work-family conflict and family-work conflict scales. *Journal of Applied Psychology, 81,* 400–410. https://doi.org/10.1037/0021-9010.81.4.400

**Work–Family Positive Spillover**

Hanson, G. C., Hammer, L. B., & Colton, C. L. (2006). Development and validation of a multidimensional scale of perceived work-family positive spillover. *Journal of Occupational Health Psychology, 11,* 249–265. https://doi.org/10.1037/1076-8998.11.3.249

**Workload**

Spector, P. E., & Jex, S. M. (1998). Developmental of four self-report measures of job stressors and strain: Interpersonal conflict at work scale, organizational constraints scale, quantitative workload inventory, and physical symptoms inventory. *Journal of Occupational Health Psychology, 3,* 356–367. https://doi.org/10.1037//1076-8998.3.4.356

Ragu-Nathan, T. S., Tarafdar, M., Ragu-Nathan, B. S., & Tu, Q. (2008). The consequences of technostress for end users in organizations: Conceptual development and empirical validation. *Information Systems Research, 19,* 417–433. https://doi.org/10.1287/isre.1070.0165

See p. 78 for instructions on how to obtain the full-sized, printable PDF.

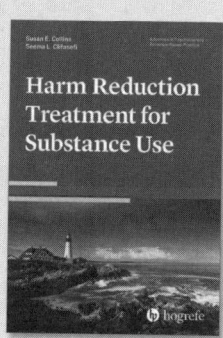
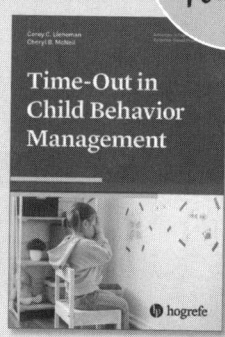
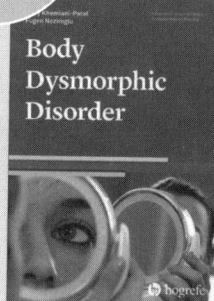
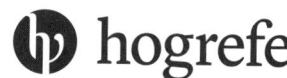

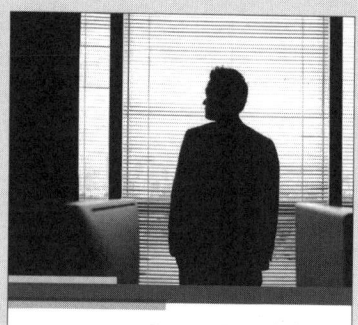
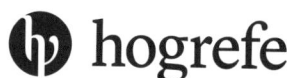